Concise Review of

CRITICAL CARE, TRAUMA AND EMERGENCY MEDICINE

A Quick Reference Guide of ICU and ER Topics

ASIF ANWAR, M.D

outskirtspress
DENVER, COLORADO

Concise Review of Critical Care, Trauma and Emergency Medicine
A Quick Reference Guide of ICU and ER Topics
All Rights Reserved.
Copyright © 2013 Asif Anwar
v2.0

Outskirts Press, Inc.
http://www.outskirtspress.com

ISBN: 978-1-4787-1608-2

Library of Congress Control Number: 2013900566

Outskirts Press and the "OP" logo are trademarks belonging to Outskirts Press, Inc.

PRINTED IN THE UNITED STATES OF AMERICA

Asif Anwar, MD, MS, FCCP
Attending Physician, Pulmonary, Critical Care and Sleep Medicine
United Hospital System, Inc., Kenosha, Wisconsin
Clinical Assistant Professor of Medicine, University of Wisconsin,
Madison-Wisconsin
Clinical Assistant Professor of Medicine, Marquette University,
Milwaukee, Wisconsin
Major, United States Air Force-R (MC) Critical Care Air Transport
Team (CCATT), & Flight Surgeon (Wisconsin Air National Guard)

This book is dedicated to my dad, Major (Retired-Army) M. Anwar, and mom, Kalsum Anwar, and to family, mentors, and the great institutions that I have been affiliated with.

I am grateful to my patients for giving me an opportunity to take care of them, learn from them, and for allowing me a chance to touch their lives.

Finally, this book is also dedicated to my wife, Dr. Khalida Anwar, and son, Sherezaad who are a constant source of inspiration in my life.

Acknowledgment

I AM GRATEFUL to my alma mater and institutions that I have been affiliated with, which include:

Military College (MCJ), LMC/SMC-UK, Northeastern Illinois University-Chicago, Morristown Memorial Hospital-University of New Jersey (UMDNJ), and Saint Louis University, Missouri. I also proudly revere my association with Lutheran General Hospital Chicago-Advocate Health Systems and Saint Luke's Medical Center-Milwaukee.

I am indebted to my colleagues, students, residents, fellows, nurses, respiratory therapists, physical therapists, and the allied health professionals who supported me during my clinical endeavors. I am indebted to United Hospital Systems Inc., especially Tom Duncan, for giving me the opportunity to be a part of a great institution and perform my military duties. I am grateful to my colleagues Dr. Mariani, Dr. Bloom, and Dr. Habel for their support of my military service.

I would like to express my appreciation for the artistic contribution of Molly Flood, BFA, the daughter of Dr. Flood, who is one of the brilliant ER physicians.

Authors and Contributors

Asif Anwar, MD, MS, FCCP

Attending Physician, Pulmonary, Critical Care and Sleep Medicine
United Hospital System, Inc., Kenosha, Wisconsin
Clinical Assistant Professor of Medicine, University of Wisconsin,
    Madison
Clinical Assistant Professor of Medicine, Marquette University,
    Milwaukee
Major (R-MC), United States Air Force-Critical Care Air Transport
    Team (CCATT),
Flight Surgeon 128th ARW, Milwaukee, WI

John O-Horo, MD

Fellow of Pulmonary, Critical Care Medicine
Mayo Clinic, Rochester Minneapolis

Ryan Servais, Pharm D

Critical Care Pharmacist
Saint Luke's Aurora Medical Center
Milwaukee, Wisconsin

Aamir Bukhari, MBA
Department of Business and Computer Information
University of Texas, Houston, Texas

Sherezaad A. Anwar
Undergraduate Student
Loyola University, Chicago, Illinois

Umer Nasim, MD
Research Assistant
Advocate Health Systems, Chicago, Illinois

Gregory Conrad, DO, Major
Attending Physician Emergency Medicine
128th ARW, Wisconsin Air National Guard, Milwaukee, Wisconsin

Jennifer A. Baughman, RN, BSN, TNS
ICU/Trauma Educator
Saint Catherine's Medical Center, Kenosha, Wisconsin

Contents

Disclaimer

THE CONTENTS OF this book are for the quick reference purpose in the field of adult Critical Care, Trauma, and Emergency Medicine.

Authors and publishers bear no responsibility for the clinical consequences resulting from the use of this reference material. Multiple sources were used during the compilation of this review. Due to the ever-changing face and practice of medicine, it is recommended that a compendium of other published material, online resources, and clinical judgment is used during the bedside clinical decision-making. Finally, this book covers the most commonly encountered clinical scenarios rather than an all-inclusive and exhaustive review of the subject matter.

Chest X-Ray Interpretation

IDENTIFICATION:

Always ensure that the reviewed image is of the correct patient, verifying date of birth with correct date and time of the imaging. This is done to avoid any confusion due to similarities in names. Sometimes multiple films are obtained on the same patient after intervention. This includes placement of a chest tube for pneumothorax, post intubation, or after a central line placement.

POSITION:

Evaluate the position in which the X-ray was obtained (e.g., posterior-anterior [PA] or anterior-posterior [AP] "portable" view). Check for incidental rotation. (Measure clavicular head distance to the imaginary midline at mid-sternum, which divides the chest into left and right half—refer to the mid-clavicular mark.) This is best described in Image 1-A, compared to a leftward rotation in Image 1-B.

Image 1-A: Centered (midline)

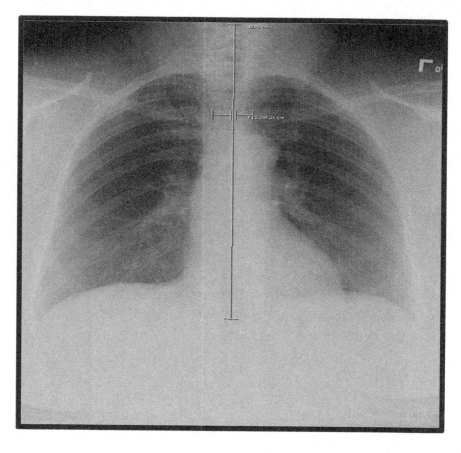

Image 1-B: Off Center (midline is towards the left)

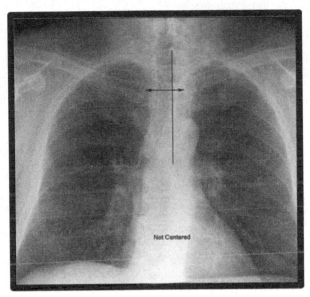

Not Centered

QUALITY OF THE FILM AND LUNG PENETRATION:

Evaluate film penetration. In a well-penetrated film the viewer should be able to see the retro-cardiac structures (i.e., inter-vertebral disc space). Both lungs should be visible with no cutoffs. Under-penetrated films would appear white or radio-opaque (compare Image 1-C with the over-penetrated film 1-D, which appears black or radiolucent). Finally, external wires should not obscure visual fields. An effort should be made to remove the extra wires (i.e., EKG leads, necklaces) from the field of imaging, as they will cast an artifactual shadow and interfere with the film interpretation.

Also discern if the image was taken on full inspiration (inhalation), such as Image 1-E, or if it was taken on expiration (exhalation), such as in Image 1-F. On a good inspiratory film, one should count eight to ten ribs.

Image 1-C: Radio-opaque (under-penetrated)
Everything appears white

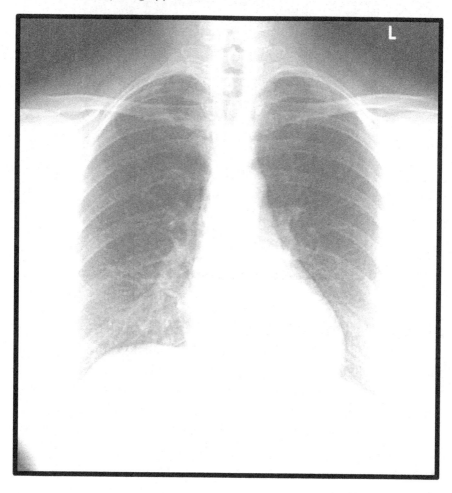

Image 1-D: Radiolucent (over-penetrated)
Everything appears black

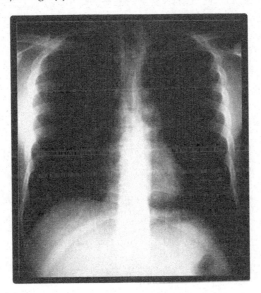

Image 1-E: Inspiratory Film

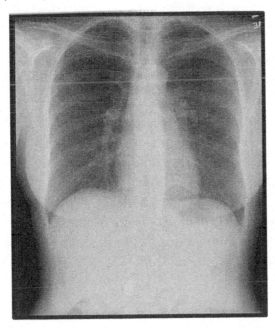

Image 1-F: Expiratory Film

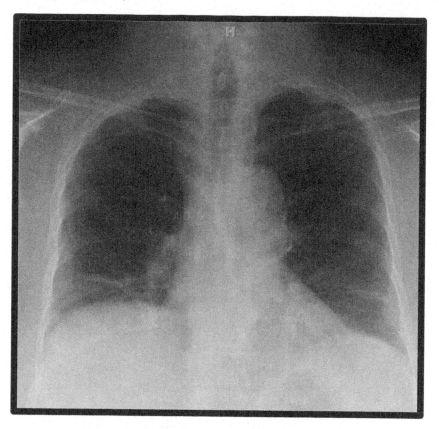

BONY ABNORMALITIES:

Evaluate images for fractures or bony abnormalities. These may appear as a loss of bony integrity or step offs at joint spaces. Thinning of bones can be a sign of osteopenia and osteoporosis, making these bones more susceptible to fracture. Osteophytes are bony protrusions that suggest degenerative joint disease. Metastatic lesions can be seen as bony abnormalities on plane films; however, bone scan or CT scan/MRI is a better diagnostic modality to look for the bony metastasis (mets).

HARDWARE:

Imaging software allows for the manipulation of radiological images. For example, the image can be inverted, which helps locate ET tubes, central lines, and feeding tubes. Endotracheal (ET) tubes should be below the clavicular heads, or three to five centimeters (cm) above the carina. Central lines should terminate at the caval-atrial junction (where superior vena cava joins the right atrium). Chest tubes are identified by radio-opaque lines and the sentinel holes (break points in the continuity of the radio-opaque line). Look for any soft tissue abnormality or presence of subcutaneous air. Nasogastric/orogastric tubes should be traceable below the diaphragm and into the gastric bubble (fundus of the stomach which casts radiolucent shadow below the left hemi-diaphragm because of presence of air), and these tubes should follow the midline. An overtly off-center NG/OG tube may be indicative of the tube being inadvertently placed in the lung. This is more common in heavily sedated, intoxicated, intubated, or elderly patients who have compromised gag and cough reflexes.

SOFT TISSUE:

Evaluate the size of heart and mediastinum, as well as look for lung opacities and fluid collections in the pericardial and pleural spaces. Tracing out to the edges of the lung markings and noting clear lines of demarcation can reveal the pneumothorax. Look for pleural abnormalities, plaques, and thickening, which can represent asbestos-related lung disease.

DIAPHRAGM:

Search for the presence of intra-abdominal free air under the diaphragm, which represents perforation of a hollow viscus or organ. This is considered a surgical emergency. Abnormalities of the diaphragmatic contour may reflect infiltrate, effusion, mass, or atelectasis. Deep sulcus (when the lateral edge of the hemi-diaphragm is deeper than the contra-lateral side) is a sign of pneumothorax. A sharp costophrenic angle represents normal shape of the diaphragm.

COMPARISON TO THE PREVIOUS IMAGE:

Major abnormalities, if stable or improved, may be of little significance. Minor abnormalities, if new, could be of greater relevance. Therefore, comparison of the films is an important aspect in the surveillance of radiological abnormalities, such as lung nodules and masses. These changes can be followed linearly over time for monitoring purposes.

COMPARE TO RADIOLOGY REPORT:

Comparing your impressions with that of a radiologist is the best way to enhance your X- ray reading skills.

MNEMONIC FOR APPROACHING CXRs (ABCDEFGHI):

A - Airway	**E** - Evaluate for effusion
B - Breathing	**F** - Foreign bodies
C - Cardiac shadow	**G** - Gastric bubble
D – Diaphragm	**H–I** - Trace from hilum through interstitium

Image 1-G: Normal Chest X-ray AP (Anteroposterior view)

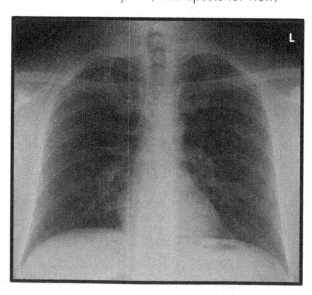

Image 1-H: Normal Chest X-ray, Lateral (Lateral view)

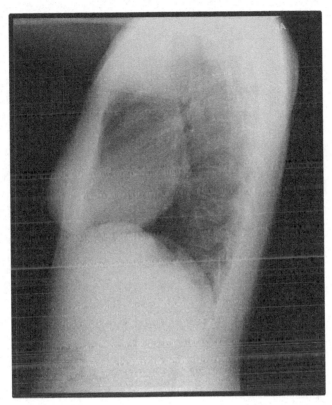

How To Evaluate A Critically Ill Patient

1) RICHMOND Approach;
Mnemonic: R-RICHMOND

- **R**espiratory
  - Lungs/airway disease, COPD
  - IPF, PFTs, ABGs, number of days on the ventilator
- **R**enal
  - Kidney function/electrolytes
  - GFR, if patient is on HD, schedule, calculate dry weight
- **I**nfectious
  - Infectious diseases/immune compromised states, i.e., HIV
  - Culture, sensitivities, antibiotics and duration of treatment
- **C**ardiac
  - Cardiac function, ejection fraction (EF-normal 55-65%)
  - Vascular function, e.g., shock state, or PAD/PVD
  - Swan-Ganz numbers or hemodynamic status, CVP
  - Fluid balance and intake/output
- **H**ematologic
  - Anemia, hypo / hyper coagulability, white cell and platelet count
  - Coumadin, aspirin, Plavix
- **M**etabolic
  - Nutrition and endocrine abnormalities, diabetes, Hb A1c
  - Pre-albumin level
- **O**ther (Oncologic / Orthopedic / Integumentary - Skin)/ OBGYN
  - Anything not fitting elsewhere
- **N**eurologic
  - Stroke/Sedation/Pain control
- **D**isposition
  - What criteria has to be satisfied for this patient to safely leave the ICU and transfer to medical/ surgical floor or discharge home/rehab/ nursing home

Systems-Based Approach

2) Head-to-Toe Approach (Alternate to R-RICHMOND):

▪ Neurologic
  – Pain/Sedation/CNS
▪ Respiratory
  – Airway/Lung Disease
▪ Cardiac
  – Fluid status, cardiac function
  – Shock States
▪ Renal/electrolyte
▪ GI/nutrition
▪ Hematologic
▪ Infectious
	▪ Integument (skin, nails, hair)
	▪ Endocrine
	  – Blood Sugar Control
	▪ Disposition
	  – What criteria must be
	    satisfied to leave ICU
	▪ Ethics
	    Code status
	  – Last family meeting
	▪ Prophylaxis
	  – DVT
	  – GI/PUD

How to Present a Patient during the "Multi-Disciplinary Rounds"

Start your presentation with the description of patient's gender, race, and co-existing medical condition pertaining to the chief complaint. For example, a 54-year-old Caucasian male with a 40-year smoking history, uncontrolled hypertension, and diabetes when presenting with crushing chest pain suggests cardiac etiology, angina, or MI, rather than an infectious cause such as pneumonia. Another example is a 74-year-old female who is a nursing home resident with advanced dementia presents with respiratory distress, fever, and hypotension. This patient's presentation points towards an infectious cause such as pneumonia or sepsis. This clinical scenario could also suggest aspiration pneumonia and is less likely related to an underlying coronary artery disease. It does not mean that this patient cannot have an underlying CAD. Perhaps further work-up may be considered in the appropriate clinical setting. Once this opening description is given, proceed with the pertinent positive and negative physical exam findings. For example, mention the cardiac rhythm such as atrial fibrillation or normal sinus rhythm, as these represent pertinent positive or pertinent negative findings, respectively. Laboratory and radiographic findings (x-ray, CT scan) specific to the disease process should be mentioned. Finally an assessment and plan for that patient, based on the systemic approach (R-Richmond or Head-to-Toe approach), should be presented. All organ systems should be mentioned in a critically ill patient, regardless if they are normal or not. This is to ensure that even smaller details are not overlooked.

Respiratory Issues in Critical Care

1. Indications for Intubation
2. Predicting a Difficult Airway: LEMON
3. Intubation: Minimal Equipment Needed
4. Anatomy of the Airway
5. Medications for Intubation
6. Methods for Intubation
7. Modes of Mechanical Ventilation
8. Ventilator-Associated Pressures
9. Re-Expansion Pulmonary Edema
10. Neurogenic Pulmonary Edema
11. Negative Pressure Pulmonary Edema (NPPE)
12. Cardiogenic Pulmonary Edema
13. Diffuse Alveolar Hemorrhage
14. Aspiration Pneumonitis
15. Pneumonitis versus Pneumonia
16. Ventilator-Induced Diaphragmatic Dysfunction (VIDD)
17. Disorders of Ventilation
18. Noninvasive Positive Pressure Ventilation (CPAP/BIPAP)
19. Pneumonia Score
20. Pneumonia Classifications
21. Ventilator-Associated Pneumonia (VAP)
22. Ventilator-Associated Tracheitis (VAT)
23. Ventilator Weaning/Liberation
24. Pneumothorax
25. Atelectasis
26. Acute Respiratory Distress Syndrome (ARDS)

27. PEEP "Recruitment"
28. ARDSnet Study
29. Prone Position Ventilation
30. Pulmonary Embolism (PE)
31. Sepsis Syndrome
32. Toxic Shock Syndrome
33. Lemierre's Disease
34. Hypoxia and its Classification
35. Decompression Sickness (DCS)

Indications for Intubation

"No set standards or guidelines define the criteria for intubation; current recommendations are based on the expert opinions and individual practices."

A SIMPLE RULE FOR INTUBATION

"If you are thinking about intubation, then you should intubate." Paul Marino Obtaining additional workup such as ABGs and CXR may be necessary as a baseline evaluation. However, waiting for the results would only delay the inevitable.

➤ **Common Reasons for Intubation:**
  ▪ **Inability to Protect the Airway**
    ▫ Trauma patient with GCS<8
    ▫ Glasgow Coma Scale (GCS) is not very predictive in non-trauma patients. It is also not a very useful tool in patients receiving sedation. Therefore clinical judgment is required, rather relying on a set of numbers.
  ▪ **Hypoxic Respiratory Failure;** Refractory to Other Measures
    ▫ Acute Respiratory Distress Syndrome (ARDS) is not an indication for Non-Invasive Positive Pressure

Ventilation (NIPPV); rather these patients should be evaluated for endotracheal intubation (conventional method) and full mechanical ventilatory support, usually on A/C mode.

- **Hyperbaric Respiratory Failure**
  - Use pH instead of carbon dioxide (CO_2) in a patient with COPD. Allowing permissive hypercapnia is an acceptable ventilatory modality. However, the pCO_2 should not exceed 90 mmHg or pH should not fall below 7.2.
- **Significant particular matter in airway;** foreign body, mucous plug, hemoptysis or hematemesis
- **Status epilepticus, status cataplecticus, or tetany**
- **Deep Sedation**
- **Surgeries/Procedures (OR setting)**
- **Increased Work of Breathing (WOB)**
  - Patients in the ER, ICU, or in the field should be evaluated for intubation and mechanical ventilatory support based on their breathing effort. These patients may be able to maintain optimal oxygen saturation and acceptable ABG numbers, but may be struggling to breathe or gasping for air. This paradoxical breathing pattern, abdomino-thoracic or "reverse breathing," can't be sustained for prolonged periods and may necessitate elective intubation and mechanical ventilation. This pattern of breathing may be more important in patients with asthma, where lack of forceful breathing efforts (shallow breathing) or a normal ABG may point towards impending respiratory failure. These patients may be seen sitting in a "tripod" position or have "guppy breathing." Also look for the signs of accessory muscle use, ala nasi (flaring of the nares), or sternocleidomastoid muscle (neck muscles) use. This effort is suggestive of respiratory distress and

should be treated with appropriate noninvasive or invasive ventilatory support.

Predicting a Difficult Airway: LEMON

➢ **Look for external factors that make airway assessment difficult:**
  ▪ Facial trauma, large incisors, facial hair, foreign body
  ▪ Large tongue (especially with Down's or Prader-Willi syndrome), angioedema, or tongue hematoma

➢ **Evaluate the 3:2:3 rule. Any of the following predict difficult intubation:**
  ▪ Incisor distance <3 fingerbreadths
  ▪ Thyromental distance <2 fingerbreadths
  ▪ Hyomental distance <3 fingerbreadths

➢ **Mallampatti >2:**
  ▪ Mallampatti I: Tonsils visible, uvula doesn't touch the tongue surface (easiest to intubate)
  ▪ Mallampatti II: Soft palate still visible, uvula touching the tongue surface
  ▪ Mallampatti III: Soft palate visible, tip of the uvula is obscured
  ▪ Mallampatti IV: Soft palate is completely obscured (most difficult to intubate)

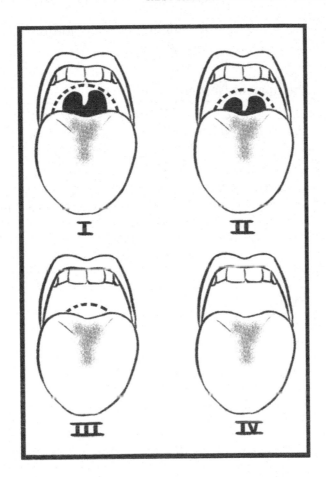

> **Obstruction:**
>   - Obesity, foreign body, previous tracheostomy, or a known history of difficult intubation
> **Neck mobility:**
>   - Cervical spine problems, C-collar (Aspen collar), or Halo
>   - Do not assess neck mobility unless C-spine injury has been clearly ruled out. Normal neck flexion is 165 to 90 degrees with a 20% loss by 75 years of age.
>   - If it is necessary to intubate patients with an unstable cervical spine, then use the in-line stabilization method. This is a two-person procedure, where one holds the neck in

a stable position, while the other performs the intubation without moving the neck.

Intubation: Equipment Needed

• Suction • Primary intubation mode and backup mode of intubation, e.g., if attempting direct laryngoscopy, have a video laryngoscope available as well • ET tube, according to the predicted size, plus one larger and smaller size • Ambu bag	• Oxygen • End tidal CO2 monitor • Drugs/medications • IV Access • Resuscitation cart ("crash cart") • Cardiac and hemodynamics monitors • Gloves/mask • Stethoscope
Difficult Intubation Kit/Cart: Glide scope Bronchoscope Bougé Intubating laryngeal mask airways (LMAs) Cricothyroidotomy/percutaneous/surgical tracheostomy tray	

Anatomy of the Airway

1) **Upper Airway**

   a. **Nose**—Roof is formed by cribriform plate of the ethmoid bone; hence with maxillofacial injury this area can be a direct portal of entry for the infectious agents into the brain. It is a highly vascular structure and therefore is susceptible to trauma or hemorrhage. It can also be a source of CSF leak, which is often associated with head trauma.

   b. **Mouth/Jaw**—Hard and soft palate forms superior surface, while oropharynx forms the posterior surface.

   c. **Nasopharynx**—Base of the skull forms the top, and soft palate forms the floor. Adenoid and lymphoid tissue can become inflamed, compromising nasal airflow.

    d. Oropharynx—Starts at the soft palate and ends at epiglottis. The tongue is the most significant structure of the oropharynx. Loss of tone of the genioglossus with anesthesia, loss of glossopharyngeal and vagus nerve function due to CNS or spinal cord injury. Tongue can cause an upper airway obstruction in patients with obstructive sleep apnea (OSA). Oropharynx can also be injured during intubation, bronchoscopy, EGD, or TEE.

2) **Middle Airway**
    a. Hypopharynx—The epiglottis is the most superior point of the hypopharynx. It forms the beginning of the esophagus at the base of the hypopharynx.
    b. Larynx—It is bound by the hypopharynx above and trachea below. Thyroid, cricoid, epiglottis, cuneiform, corniculate, and arytenoid cartilages form the main skeleton of the larynx.
    c. Trachea—Averages 15 cm in length and is made up of C-shaped cartilaginous rings anteriorly and membranous/muscular part posteriorly. Microscopically it has ciliated epithelium. Carina is located at fourth thoracic vertebrae.

3) **Lower Airway**
    a. Right main-stem is at a less acute angle to the trachea; therefore, foreign objects and aspiration contents land into right main-stem bronchus.

Medications for Intubation

1. **Topical**
    a. Lidocaine 1-4%, nebulized, atomized, or instilled, with or without epinephrine can anesthetize nasal passage and reduce trauma/bleeding during intubations or procedures such as bronchoscopies.
    b. Sub-laryngeal anesthesia may compromise the cough reflex, and increase risk of aspiration, but also may blunt vasovagal response. 4% trans-tracheal lidocaine may be

atomized or instilled topically to achieve an optimal anesthetic effect.

2. **General anesthesia** can be used with induction agents
   a. **Thiopental**
      i. Dose: 2.5-4.5 mg/kg
      ii. Onset: 20-50 seconds
      iii. Side effect: Hypotension
   b. **Propofol (Diprivan)**
      i. Dose 1.0-2.5 mg/kg
      ii. Onset: Less than a minute
      iii. Side effects: Hypotension, burning sensation with injection
   c. **Midazolam**
      i. Dose: 0.02-0.20 mg/kg
      ii. Onset 30-60 seconds
      iii. Side effects: Hypotension
   d. **Ketamine**
      i. Dose 0.5-2.0 mg/kg
      ii. Onset 30-60 seconds
      iii. Side effects: Increase intracranial pressure and increase secretions
      iv. Benefit: Hemodynamic stability
   e. **Etomidate**
      i. Dose: 0.2-0.3 mg/kg
      ii. Onset: 20-50 seconds
      iii. Side effects: Pain on injection, adrenal insufficiency
      iv. Benefits: Cardio protective profile
   f. **Paralytics (Neuromuscular blocking agents)**
      □ **Succinylcholine**
         i. Dose: 1-2 mg/kg
         ii. Onset: 45-60 seconds
         iii. Side effects: Hyperkalemia, increased intragastric pressure, increased intracranial pressure
         iv. Can cause malignant hyperthermia

▫ **Rocuronium**
  i. Dose: 0.6-1.0 mg/kg
  ii. Onset: 60-90 seconds

Methods for Intubation

Method	Pros	Cons
Direct laryngoscopy	High rate of success Fewer traumas/bleeding Low Incidence of sinusitis	Dental trauma Cervical trauma Oral hygiene Tube biting
Nasotracheal	Free access to mouth Stability No tube biting Can be done blindly	Sinusitis Bleeding Cannot be used in facial, head, and neck trauma
Fiber optic	Easier and direct visualization of the vocal cords Good for traditionally difficult airways Higher success in awake patients Distance between the end of ET tube and carina can be measured	Difficulty visualizing in presence of secretions or blood
Laryngeal Mask Airway (LMA)	Always achievable Single-handed Patient can be intubated	Does not protect against aspiration
Tracheostomy/ Crico thyroidotomy	Ideal when there is an upper airway obstruction caused by trauma, burns, swelling	Damage to the anterior neck structures, and bleeding

Modes of Mechanical Ventilation

➢ **Control:** Breaths entirely defined by the clinician

➢ **Assist:** Ventilator reduces the work of breathing due to the spontaneous breaths. Patient is allowed to breathe over the set ventilatory rate and tidal volume. However, the patient is assured a pre-set tidal volume and a set respiratory rate.

➢ **Triggers:**
- **Time-Cycled:** Breath triggered every few seconds at a set rate
- **Pressure:** Particular negative pressure triggers breath
- **Flow:** Intake flow triggers breath

➢ **Control Variables:**
- **Volume:** Pre-set target volume is delivered, pressure fluctuates
- **Pressure:** Target peak pressure ends the breath, volume fluctuates

➢ **Other Variables:**
- **FiO2:** Fraction of inspired oxygen

Graphical Representation of Pressure Over Time

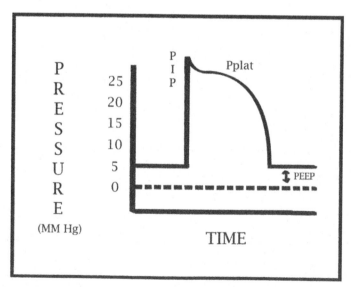

Ventilator-Associated Pressures

➤ **Peak Inspiratory Pressure (PIP):**
- Reflects the pressure in the upper airways, including the pressure in the ventilatory circuit and tubing
- It is the highest pressure recorded during breath delivery, correlates with large airway resistance
- Elevated in patients with bronchospasm, obstruction, secretions, and water condensation in the ventilator's circuit / tubing *obstructive*
- Target PIP should be less than 30 mmHg
- The pressure should decrease after bronchodilator treatment if bronchospasm was the underlying etiology

➤ **Plateau Pressure (Pplat):**
- This pressure translates the pressure within the lung parenchyma
- Stable pressure is reached once breath is delivered if an inspiratory hold is applied. It is a measure of small airway resistance
- Elevated in conditions causing lung stiffening, i.e., ARDS, pneumonia, pulmonary contusions *restrictive*
- Target Pplat should be less than 30 mmHg

➤ **Positive End Expiratory Pressure (PEEP):**
- Pressure in the alveoli at the end-expiration, which is necessary to keep the alveoli open at end of each breath
- This is usually applied to the ventilator settings to assist in the delivery of oxygen and keeping the alveoli open at the end-exhalation
- PEEP is usually initiated at 5 mmHg, but can be adjusted according to the oxygenation and the FiO_2 requirements. (Refer to the suggested FiO_2/PEEP ratios in the ARDS section)

➤ **Auto-PEEP:**
- High PEEP generated in the alveoli in COPD patients that can be assessed by reviewing the ventilatory loops/graphs

- The PEEP may be adjusted to compensate for the auto-PEEP
- If difficult to maintain optimal ventilation due to an auto-PEEP, then the ventilator should be disconnected from the ET tube. The excess trapped air should be allowed to escape and the patient reattached to the ventilator

Re-expansion Pulmonary Edema

➤ **Definition:** Rapid development of bilateral (R>L) infiltrative changes in the lung shortly after drainage of a large and usually long-standing pleural effusion
➤ **Etiology/Risk Factors:**
- Mechanical lung injury
- Free radical injury
- Increased vascular permeability
- Young age

➤ **Mortality:** 19%
➤ **Treatment:** Supportive care
➤ **Drainage Method:**
- Pleural manometry should not be more than negative 20 mmHg (measured by a pressure monitoring of the pleural fluids).
- Remove only 1 to 1.5 L of the pleural fluid at any given time provided the patient does not develop symptoms of chest pain, cough, or dyspnea. However, chronic large volume pleural effusion can be drained without any complications if patient remains asymptomatic and hemodynamically stable during the fluid removal.

➤ **Large volumes of pleural fluid can be drained if:**
- A mediastinal shift is present
- The patient remains asymptomatic during the drainage process
- There is a chronic large pleural effusion causing respiratory distress

Neurogenic Pulmonary Edema

➤ **Definition:** It is a rapid development of bilateral pulmonary edema secondary to any central nervous system (CNS) etiology. This often requires ventilatory support.

➤ **Diagnosis:**
- Absence of cardiac and pulmonary diseases such as CHF or pneumonia
- Radiological evidence of bilateral pulmonary edema

➤ **Etiology/Risk Factors:**
- Lung injury associated with stroke (CVA), trauma, or other CNS catastrophe
- Surge of catecholamine release is suspected as the underlying pathology

➤ **Mortality:** Unknown

➤ **Treatment:**
- Supportive care
- Phentolamine infusion has shown some promise in reducing the pulmonary edema in susceptible patients.

Negative Pressure Pulmonary Edema (NPPE)

➤ **Definition:**
- It is non-cardiogenic pulmonary edema that results from an abrupt upper airway obstruction. This obstruction can be caused by an extreme bronchospasm (in susceptible individuals post extubation), during an asthma exacerbation, or after strangulation (homicide, or suicide by hanging).
- Frank hemorrhage or hemoptysis may occur.

➤ **Pathogenesis:**
- Development of pulmonary edema caused by sudden fluid accumulation. This results from the vigorous inspiratory effort against an obstructed airway.
- Venous return is increased.
- Increased hydrostatic pressure and capillary leak may occur.

- Increased capillary leak results in the development of pulmonary edema and hemorrhage (pink frothy sputum).
- Right ventricular distension or strain pattern may be caused by the elevated right heart pressure.
- Leftward shift of the intraventricular septum because of the elevated right-sided pressures
- Decreased left ventricular compliance
- Increased left ventricular end-diastolic pressure (LVEDP)

➢ **Clinical:**
- Dyspnea
- Hypoxia
- Crackles on the lung exam
- Pink frothy sputum or bloody sputum
- Diffuse infiltrates or pulmonary vascular congestion on the CXR

➢ **Supportive:**
- Oxygen and mechanical ventilatory support
- Bronchodilators treatment when bronchospasm is suspected or noticed
- Removal of the foreign object if it is obstructing the airway

Cardiogenic Pulmonary Edema

➢ **Definition:** Severe pulmonary edema secondary to left ventricular dysfunction

➢ **Pathogenesis:**
Pulmonary vascular congestion caused by an increased hydrostatic pressure. Cardiac diseases are the usual suspect. Clinically it may present as chest pain or shortness of breath.

➢ **Clinical Presentation:**
- Bilateral pulmonary edema or pleural effusions
- Patient has shortness of breath or chest pain
- There is often an evidence or a history of coronary artery disease

- Patient's history may reveal either noncompliance with the medications, diuretics, or dietary indiscretion, high-salt diet, "Thanksgiving Syndrome."

➢ **Chest X-ray:**
- Presents as pulmonary vascular congestion, with the "butterfly" pattern, which is also referred to as "bat wing appearance." There may also be bilateral symmetrical pleural effusion.
- There is bilateral symmetrical pulmonary vascular congestion with predilection towards the lung apices.
- The term "cephalization" is often used to describe this pattern of apical pulmonary vascular congestion.

➢ **Diagnosis:**
- Diagnosis is based on the clinical context and is evident by a CXR or the lab findings, i.e., elevated BNP or troponins.

➢ **Treatment:**
- Treatment is directed towards management of the underlying coronary artery disease. There is an immediate relief of symptoms after diuretics or giving after-load reducers, i.e., ACE-I or ARB. Venodilators such as nitroglycerin also help alleviate the symptoms of shortness of breath and chest pain in these patients.

Diffuse Alveolar Hemorrhage

➢ **Definition:**
- Bleeding in the lung and alveoli, which presents as hemoptysis or frank hemorrhage

➢ **Etiology:**
- Immune-mediated phenomenon, Wegener's Granulomatosis (WG), Goodpasture's Syndrome (GPS), or Hypersensitivity Pneumonitis (HSP)
- It is typically not associated with chronic interstitial changes

> **Symptoms/Signs:**
  - Respiratory insufficiency or failure, requiring ventilatory support
  - Hemoptysis, which may be massive (>300 cc) or sub-massive (<300 cc)
> **Diagnosis:**
  - New infiltrate on the CXR or CT scan
  - Pathology/histology shows leukocytoclastic vasculitis and inflammatory cells
> **Prognosis:**
  - Mortality 50-70%
  - Worse in women
  - Higher acuity of the disease on its initial presentation is associated with worst prognosis and outcomes
  - Bleak prognosis for the patients who require mechanical ventilation
> **Diagnosis:**
  - Bronchoscopy with progressively increasing bloody fluid on the serial bronchoalveolar lavage (BAL) specimens
> **Treatment:**
  - Steroids, usually in the stress doses, are required 2mg/kg preferably IV route
  - Immunosuppression
    □ Azathioprine
    □ Cyclosporine (avoid in pregnancy)

Aspiration Pneumonitis

> **Definition:** Acute lung injury (ALI) following aspiration of the oral and gastric contents (contents are acidic with a pH<4)
> **Risk Factors:**
  - Drug overdose/alcohol/seizure
  - Nursing home, elderly, mentally challenged, or institutionalized patients
  - Psychiatric medications such as Haldol and Risperdal are

associated with high risk of aspiration due to weakness of the deglutition muscles.

- Large volume aspiration is usually witnessed.

➤ **Treatment:**
- Antibiotics are generally not indicated within the first 48 hours of aspiration.
- If the patient is at a high risk for developing pneumonia, i.e., patient with alcoholism or poor dental hygiene, then antibiotic use may be warranted. These antimicrobials should cover for the oral microbial flora, i.e., anaerobes.
- Steroids offer no additional benefit in this clinical context.
- Bronchoscopy is not typically indicated acutely, unless there is aspiration of solid food particles, foreign body, or there is an airway obstruction. NIPPV (CPAP/BIPAP) is relatively contraindicated with the patients who are at a risk for aspiration.

Pneumonitis versus Pneumonia

PNEUMONITIS	PNEUMONIA
• Aspiration of gastric contents	• Colonized oropharyngeal materials
• Acute lung injury (ALI) or Acute respiratory distress syndrome (ARDS) from the gastric acid aspiration	• Inflammation from the bacterial products/toxins
• Initially indistinguishable from an infection	• Gram positive cocci (GPC), gram negative rods (GNR), and anaerobes from the oropharyngeal flora
• Predisposed by decreased loss of consciousness (LOC) and inability to protect one's airway	• Predisposed by dysphagia
• More often in young patient with a drug overdose	• More often in elderly patients who have dysphagia
• Respiratory distress usually ensues within 2-5 hours after the witnessed aspiration event	• Tachypnea or cough may be the presenting symptom
	• There is a prodrome of systemic inflammatory response syndrome (SIRS) or sepsis

Ventilator-Induced Diaphragmatic Dysfunction (VIDD)

➢ **Definition:**
- Diaphragmatic muscle abnormality induced by mechanical ventilation

➢ **Pathogenesis:**
- Associated with high-level assist control ventilation
- Atrophy of the respiratory muscles may occur
- There is loss of myofibril, which is caused by the oxidative stress
- There is an increased muscle protein breakdown, which is further exacerbated by the sepsis and the associated catabolic process
- It can develop within 24 hours of mechanical ventilation
- Other causes of muscle injury include:
  □ Critical illness neuropathy
  □ Steroid-induced myopathy
  □ Neuromuscular blocking agents (NMB)
  □ Co-morbid clinical conditions, muscle injury, GBS, MG, etc.

➢ **Treatment:**
- Avoid prolonged and high-level mechanical ventilatory support.
- Allow for the spontaneous breathing effort (pressure support ventilation) or "vent weaning."
- Decrease or discontinue the use of steroids and neuromuscular agents as soon as it is clinically feasible.
- Early mobilization, which is often accomplished with the "daily sedation vacation," helps reduce number of days on the ventilator and length of ICU stay (LOS).

Disorders of Ventilation

➢ **Central control:**
- Idiopathic or primary central hypoventilation (Ondine's Curse). A congenital abnormality caused by a defect in

the PHOX2-B gene
- Central sleep apnea (CSA) with Cheyenne-Stokes respiration (CSR) is caused by CHF, CVA, and renal failure
- Narcotics/sedative overdose
- Intracranial pathology (medullary disease), e.g., tumor, infarct (bulbar infarct)
- Hypothyroidism
- Metabolic acidosis, renal failure, or infections
- Rabies (rare cause)

➤ **Motor neuron:**
- Spinal cord injury
- Disorder of anterior horn cells, e.g., amyotrophic lateral sclerosis (ALS) or Lou Gehrig's disease, poliomyelitis
- Tetanus

➤ **Peripheral neuropathy:**
- Guillain-Barré syndrome (GBS)
- Critical illness polyneuropathy
- Critical illness myopathy

➤ **Neuromuscular junction:**
- Myasthenia gravis (MG)
- Eaton-Lambert syndrome (ELS)
- Organophosphate poisoning (accidental in farming industry or drug overdose with a suicidal or homicidal intent)
- Botulism (canned food or stored honey)
- Neuromuscular (NM) blockade with a non-depolarizing agent

Noninvasive Positive Pressure Ventilation (CPAP/BIPAP)

➤ **Definition:** This is a mode of mechanical ventilation where the patient is not intubated with the endotracheal tube (ET tube). Usually a face mask suffices as an interface for the delivery of positive pressure ventilation.

➤ **Types:**
- CPAP (Continuous Positive Pressure Ventilation): one

constant pressure is applied throughout the respiration, i.e., both inspiration and expiration.

- BIPAP (Bi-level Positive Pressure Ventilation): a mode of ventilation when two different pressures (IPAP/EPAP) are applied during respiration.
- The IPAP (Inspiratory Positive Airway) is the pressure applied during the inspiration and mimics the tidal volume (TV) on conventional ventilators. It should be targeted towards the ideal body weight. The range for the TV is 6-8 cc/kg. The usual starting IPAP is 10 cm H20, which is adjusted to the target TV.
- EPAP (Expiratory Positive Airway Pressure) is the pressure applied at exhalation phase of respiration, and mimics the PEEP on the conventional ventilator. It is usually started at 5 cm H20, and may be adjusted for optimal oxygenation.
- If PCO2 is increased on the ABGs, IPAP should be increased. On the other hand, EPAP and FiO2 fraction can be increased if the oxygen saturation—i.e., PaO2, or SpO2 (pulse ox)—is low. The difference in the EPAP and IPAP is more important than either of the pressures alone, i.e., IPAP and EPAP. This difference of the IPAP and EPAP is the pressure support.

➢ **Relative Contraindications:**
  - Unconscious or obtunded patient who is unable to protect the airway
  - Facial trauma, facial hair (mask does not fit properly and can cause significant air leak)
  - Pneumonia
  - ARDS

➢ **Indications:**
  - COPD/Asthma exacerbation
  - Pulmonary edema (decompensated CHF)
    - BIPAP/CPAP should be used as a bridge to either stability or failure of the respiratory status. In either case

it is a short-term modality of treatment in patients with respiratory distress. If patient doesn't tolerate or fails the noninvasive positive pressure therapy (CPAP/ BIPAP), then conventional modes of ventilatory failure such as intubation and mechanical ventilation should be initiated.

Pneumonia Score
> **CURB 65:**
>   □ Confusion
>   □ Uremia (BUN>20)
>   □ Respiratory rate (>30)
>   □ Blood pressure (diastolic <65)
>   □ 65 (age)
>   ▪ Each parameter gets a point
>   ▪ Score >3 is associated with a 20% mortality, and requires in-patient treatment
> **Factors associated with low risk of failure:**
>   ▪ Flu vaccination
>   ▪ COPD (since symptoms are often recognized and treated early on)
>   ▪ Use of quinolones with anti-pneumococcal activity
> **Factors associated with high risk of failure:**
>   ▪ Liver disease
>   ▪ High pneumonia risk score
>   ▪ Leukopenia
>   ▪ Multi-lobar infiltrate
>   ▪ Pleural effusion
>   ▪ Radiographic signs of cavitation
> **Treatment:** Combination of antibiotics and other supportive modalities, i.e., supplemental oxygen or mechanical ventilation with NIPPV (CPAP/BIPAP) vs. intubation. Antibiotics should be initiated as soon as possible, as delaying the administration of empiric antibiotics affects the mortality. The

suggested "door to needle time" should be within two hours of arriving in the ER. Concordant antibiotic therapy (later cultures results show microorganisms were susceptible to the initial empiric antibiotics administered) confers better survival as compared with discordant antibiotic therapy (bugs resistant to the empiric course of antibiotics).

PNEUMONIA ON CT CHEST (Air-Bronchogram in the right lung)

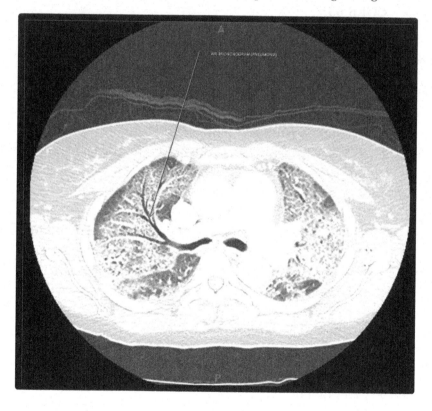

CXR-Pneumonia

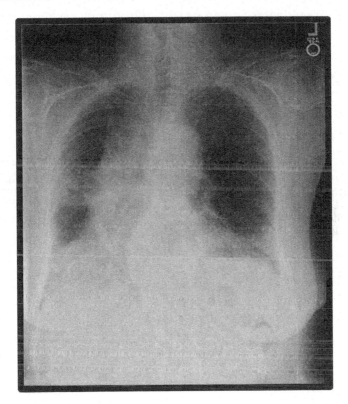

Pneumonia Classifications

A: Community-Acquired Pneumonia (CAP):

This is defined as respiratory infection acquired while residing in the community setting. For example, a patient coming from home with new pneumonia symptoms would be considered as having a CAP.

- Bacteria: Typical: Streptococcus (most common), staphylococcus (MSSA or MRSA); Atypical: Mycoplasma, legionella, and chlamydia; Unusual: Fungus in immune-compromised individuals; Influenza: A&B
- Viruses: Rhinovirus, orthomyxovirus, RSV, metapneumovirus

B: Healthcare-Acquired Pneumonia (HCAP):

Any evidence of new pneumonia symptoms acquired while in contact with the healthcare setting, within the past thirty days of symptoms' onset. This includes being in a nursing home, a recent visit to the ER, or hospitalization.

- Bacteria: Strep, staph (MRSA), pseudomonas
- Viruses

C: Pneumonia in an Immune-compromised Host:

New respiratory symptoms in a patient with history of an underlying cancer are suggestive of pneumonia. Patient on high-dose steroids or immunomodulating drugs are also considered immune-compromised. Pneumonia in these patients may be caused by:

- Bacteria
- Viruses
- Fungus

D: Endemic/Pandemic Pneumonia:

- Pneumonia caused by viral agents due to antigenic shift or drift. Spanish flu of 1918 is an example of pandemic infection.
- Bird flu or severe acute respiratory syndrome (SARS) virus

E: Aspiration Pneumonia:

- Oral/Gastric contents
- Foreign body

F: Miscellaneous Causes of Pneumonia:

- Pneumonitis caused by oral/gastric aspiration is a form of chemical pneumonitis
- Hypersensitivity pneumonitis (HSP)
- Interstitial lung disease (ILD)
- Ventilator-associated pneumonia (VAP)

Ventilated-Associated Pneumonia (VAP)

Definition: Pneumonia in a mechanically ventilated patient after being on the ventilator for more than 48 hours

Diagnosis: Clinical microbiology specimens obtained from the tracheal aspirate or bronchoalveolar lavage (BAL) may be suggestive but not crucial for the diagnosis of VAP.

➤ **Pathogenesis:**

It is caused by aspiration of the stagnant upper respiratory secretions, which harbor both normal and pathologic flora from the upper respiratory tract. There is an increased risk if the cuff of the endotracheal (ET) tube is deflated without prior aggressive suctioning of the stagnant subglottic secretions. There are some silent secretions that are aspirated into the lung from above the endotracheal cuff. Since it is not a perfect barrier to prevent the downstream flow of secretions, there is a potential for VAT/VAP.

➤ **Treatment:**

- Empiric antibiotics, which cover pseudomonas, MRSA, and other microorganisms associated with the healthcare-acquired infections.
- Application of the specialized endotracheal tubes, which apply constant suctioning, i.e., subglottic suctioning ET tubes. These tubes are a good prophylactic measure to prevent VAP.
- Avoid cuff deflation or breaking the integrity of the closed ventilator circuit. Therefore, in-line suctioning is recommended rather than disconnecting the ventilator and performing endotracheal deep suctioning.

➤ **Prevention:**

- "VAP bundle" includes:
  - Keeping head of the bed elevated >30 degrees (unless C/I)
  - Daily sedation vacation
  - DVT prophylaxis
  - GI prophylaxis (which prevents DVT/PE and GI bleeds)
  - Oral care with chlorhexidine

Ventilated-Associated Tracheitis (VAT)

Definition: Infection of the upper airways, trachea, or bronchioles that occurs in the mechanically ventilated patient after 48 hours of intubation. There is no evidence of pneumonia on the CXR.

Diagnosis: It is a clinical diagnosis. Microbiology specimens obtained from the tracheal aspirate or bronchoalveolar lavage (BAL) may be suggestive but not critical for the diagnosis of VAT.

Treatment: Fairly similar to the VAP, as far as choice of initial antibiotic regimen is concerned. There is less morbidity or mortality associated with VAT than VAP.

Ventilator Weaning/Liberation

➢ Make sure that the primary reason for which the patient was intubated has been resolved. Various kinds of shock, pneumonia, and cardiac causes can lead to respiratory failure. Then apply the acronym **"MOVE"** to assess for weaning. Every criteria has to be met before any extubation attempt:

- **M** – Mental Status (patient is able to follow simple commands)
- **O** – Oxygenation (requiring 0.4% FiO2 [40 percent or less oxygen])
- **V** – Ventilation (RSBI* should be less than 105)
- **E** – Expectoration of secretions (should require suctioning less than every four hours)
  - **A cuff leak test** should also be performed to assess for the airway swelling around the ET tube. If there is no cuff leak after the balloon is deflated, this reflects bronchospasm or edema around the endotracheal tube. This condition may require steroids before extubation is attempted. Auscultate the neck after the extubation to listen for "stridor," which is heard as a loud pitch noise on inspiration. This represents bronchospasm and may require nebulized racemic epinephrine treatments, which can be repeated a few

times. Resistant cases may benefit from heliox, which provides a linear oxygen flow (due to helium), compared with the regular oxygen, which has turbulent flow pattern due to the presence of nitrogen gas. If all fails, patient will need re-intubation. If there is severe bronchospasm and the conventional method of intubation has failed, then emergent cricothyroidotomy or tracheotomy may be needed.

➤ **RSBI** – Rapid Shallow Breathing Index:
This number is obtained by dividing the respiratory rate by the tidal volume in liters, expressed in points. For example, if the tidal volume is 500 ml, it is expressed as 0.5 liters. If the respiratory rate is 20, then the RSBI would be 20/0.5=40. It is an excellent number to consider in order to extubate the patient, provided all other weaning parameters are met. An index (RSBI) of less than 105 is an acceptable number for extubation. For the ease of memorization, RSBI less than a 100 would suffice for extubation. The lower the RSBI, the better the chances of a successful extubation. The RSBI is more reflective and predictive of successful extubation if the maneuver is performed while the patient is off sedation and the weaning trial is performed while on a minimal pressure support and PEEP. Pressure support of five and a PEEP of five are sufficient during this "weaning trial" since some ventilatory support is needed to overcome the resistance of the tubing. A twenty-minute spontaneous breathing trial is as good as a two-hour spontaneous breathing trial. Longer weaning trials can cause undue stress on the patient and may result in fatigue and increase the risk of re-intubation. Age-old weaning parameters such as negative inspiratory force (NIF) are less predictable and reliable markers for a successful extubation.

Pneumothorax

➢ **Definition:** A collection of air in the pleural space or around the lungs. In simple terms it is collapse of the lung, which is unable to re-expand with spontaneous breaths.

➢ **Etiology:**

(a) **Iatrogenic:** This may occur following invasive procedures, i.e., insertion of central line (central venous catheter) in the internal jugular, subclavian vein, or after a PICC line placement. Thoracentesis can cause an iatrogenic pneumothorax. Patients may return from the OR with chest tubes after cardiothoracic surgeries. It may also occur during or after an intubation attempt, but this is rare.

(b) **Traumatic:** After motor vehicle accident, or blunt injury to the chest wall

(c) **Spontaneous:** In patients with underlying lung disease, i.e., emphysema/COPD, or in young asthenic, tall, thin, otherwise healthy males without any obvious lung pathology

(d) **Unusual diseases:** Catamenial disease, lymphangio-lyomatosis (LAM), alpha 1-anti-trypsin deficiency

(e) **Tension Pneumothorax:** Even though not a separate category, it can result from any of the above-mentioned etiologic factors. It pushes the vital mediastinal structures such as the heart and associated vascular structures towards the opposite side of the pneumothorax, causing a mediastinal shift. Tracheal deviation occurs opposite of the pneumothorax. The patient may also have jugular vein distention (JVD). This results in hemodynamic compromise, requiring emergent treatment, i.e., needle thoracentesis followed by a chest tube placement.

➢ **Diagnosis:**

Clinical signs and symptoms, i.e., breathing difficulties, chest pain, absent breath sounds on the affected side, deviation of the trachea, and a hyper-resonant percussion note may be observed.

➤ **Treatment:**
  ▪ Emergent needle thoracentesis
  ▪ Chest tube insertion follows the needle decompression (ranges from 16F to 38F)
  ▪ VATS/thoracotomy (in few complicated cases, i.e., bullous COPD)
  ▪ Observation for an asymptomatic spontaneous pneumothorax, with less than 20% pneumothorax on CXR
  ▪ When planning to discontinue the chest tube, it should be clamped for some time, and CXR repeated to ascertain that the pneumothorax has resolved.

MINIMAL LEFT APICAL PNEUMOTHORAX
(Difficult to appreciate on the CXR)

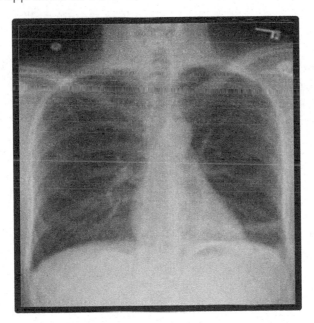

CT scan of the chest confirming the CXR finding of left pneumothorax

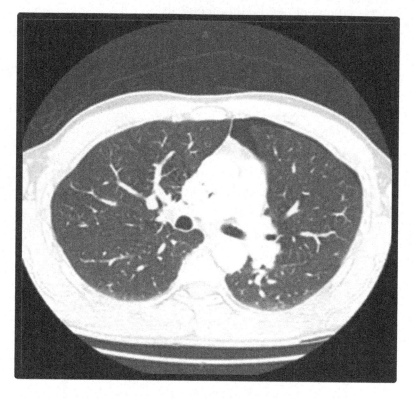

Moderate-size left pneumothorax on CT scan

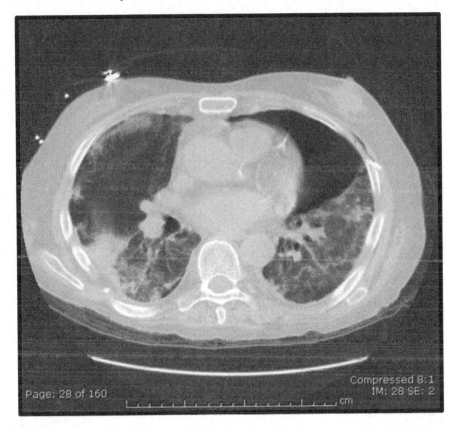

Moderate Right Lung Pneumothorax (CXR)

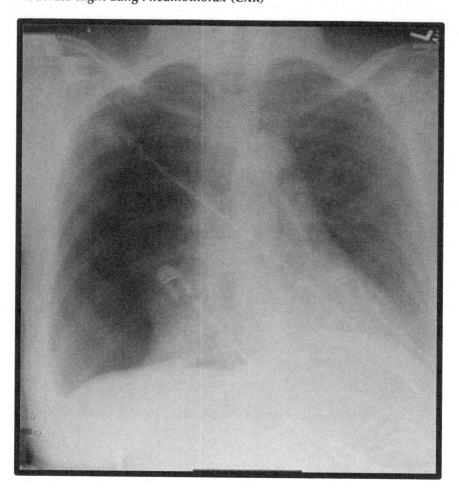

Right Pneumothorax-Arrows

(After RIJ line placement)

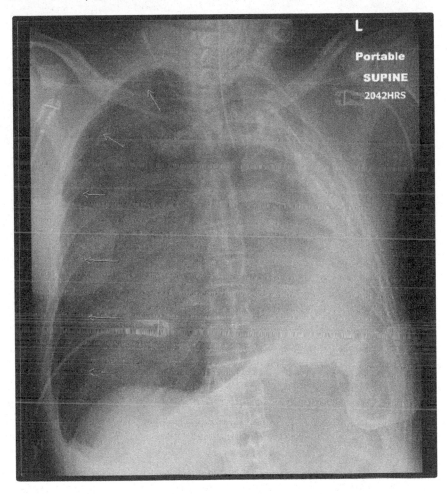

Discoid Atelectasis (Right Lower Lobe of the Lung)

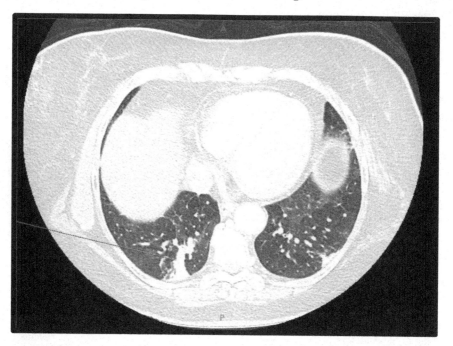

Atelectasis

> **Definition:**

It is defined as collapse of a portion of or the entire lung. Atelectasis is usually associated with some degree of volume loss of the lung.

> **Types:**

- **Obstructive (most common) and Non-Obstructive Atelectasis**

  The air in the alveoli and respiratory bronchioles is re-absorbed due to the obstruction. Common causes of obstructive atelectasis are:

- Tumor
- Foreign body
- Mucous plugging

- Shallow breathing in the post-operative period may result in collapse of dependent airway lung zones
- Severe bronchospasm

➢ **Classification according to the radiological appearance (CXR)**
- Discoid-like atelectasis
- Disc-like or Plate-like atelectasis
- Band-like atelectasis
- Rounded atelectasis

➢ **Treatment**
- Prevention is the most important factor
- Treatment of the underlying cause, I.e., removal of the foreign body or secretions
- Supplemental oxygen
- Early ambulation
- Pain control, which will prevent the shallow breathing due to "splinting"
- Bronchodilator treatments will help relieve bronchospasm
- Incentive spirometry (IS) in patients who are awake and cooperative
- Use of intermittent positive pressure ventilation (IPPV) or EZ PAP in weak, obtunded, or uncooperative patients
- Noninvasive ventilation with CPAP/BIPAP may be needed in some cases
- "Vest therapy" with Mucomyst/Pulmozyme in patients with mucous plugs, especially in cystic fibrosis (CF) or bronchiectasis
- Chest physical therapy
- Bronchoscopy may be needed in patients with respiratory compromise, especially when there is collapse of an entire lung due to mucous plug

ARDS (Acute Respiratory Distress Syndrome)
➢ **Definition:** It is an acute and diffuse inflammatory lung injury, associated with increased vascular permeability. ARDS is

characterized by stiffening of the lungs. It may be a continuation of the acute lung injury (ALI), which is often the first step in the inflammatory process and takes place as a consequence of various pathology processes such as infection or trauma.

➢ **ALI:** This kind of lung injury may present as a radiological abnormality on the CXR or CT scan. There is resultant hypoxia, with the P/F ratio of 200-300. There should be absence of the underlying cardiogenic pulmonary edema or the PCWP should be less than 18. However, in the new classification, the pulmonary artery wedge pressure criterion has been removed. Hence, hydrostatic edema in the form of cardiac failure or fluid overload states may coexist with ARDS.

➢ **ARDS: The Newer and the Refined (Berlin Definition and categories)**

CATEGORY	HYPOXIA LEVEL	DAYS ON VENT	MORTALITY
MILD	P/F ratio 200-300	5	27%
MOD	P/F ratio 100-200	7	32%
SEVERE	P/F ratio <100	9	45%

P/F Ratio: Ratio obtained by dividing the PaO_2 (partial pressure of oxygen) divided by the FiO_2 (Fraction of Inspired Oxygen). Normal P/F ratio is >300

➢ **Etiology:**

Infection: Primary lung infection, i.e., pneumonia and sepsis vs. infection from any other source (skin and soft tissue infections)

Trauma: Direct pulmonary contusion, chest trauma, near drowning, inhalation of toxic gases

Pancreatitis: Release of the pro-inflammatory cytokines and activated trypsin. Trauma is one of the most common noninfectious causes of ARDS/ALI

Medication/Toxin induced: Overdose of heroin or crack cocaine

> **Mechanism of Lung Injury:**
> **Baro-trauma:** Increased positive ventilatory pressure, i.e., PIP, Pplat, or PEEP
> **Volu-trauma:** Increased volume (Increased mortality noticed during the ARDSnet study). Therefore 6-8 cc/kg/ideal body weight should be used to calculate the TV. Delivery of high TV >10cc/kg has been associated with an increased mortality
> **Atelecto-trauma:** Caused by various pathologies leading to atelectasis
> **Bio-trauma:** Effects of drugs, overdose, and Inhalational injuries
> - These factors may be mutually exclusive or may coexist in same patient.

> **Direct versus Indirect ARDS (Another way to look at ARDS):**

DIRECT ARDS	INDIRECT ARDS
Pneumonia Aspiration Inhalational injury Chest trauma Lung contusions	Multiple trauma Shock Massive blood transfusion >10 u Sepsis Pancreatitis Post cardiopulmonary bypass High volume crystalloid infusion

> **Clinical Implications of Direct versus Indirect ARDS:**

DIRECT ARDS	INDIRECT ARDS
Consolidation on the affected site Normal chest wall mechanics Limited response to PEEP or prone position ventilation	Diffuse interstitial edema pattern Atelectasis of the dependent lung Good response to PEEP or prone position ventilation

> **Pathogenesis:** The initial injury leads to the release of cytokines and other pro-inflammatory mediators. This results in

the capillary leak, pulmonary edema, and hypoxia. The end result is "stiff" lungs, which are less pliable and less expandable during respiration.

➢ **Treatment:**

Lung Protective Strategy is the application of the low tidal volume ventilation strategy using 6-8 cc/kg ideal body weight for the determination of the tidal volume. Using a relatively low TV, but providing higher PEEP achieves this goal. There is a significant survival benefit by using the low volume strategy. This is accomplished by permitting a relatively high PCO2, and accepting low pH in turn, therefore allowing a relative respiratory acidotic state. This method of ventilation is termed "permissive hypercapnia" (pH >7.2 is acceptable range).

Acute Respiratory Distress Syndrome

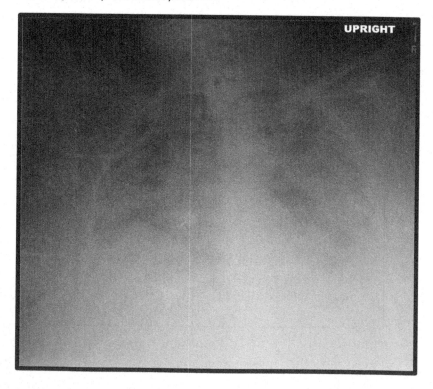

"TO PEEP OR NOT TO PEEP"

➤ **Recruitment:**

It is the application of higher and incremental PEEP to help improve the opening of the atelectatic portions of the lung. It is like inflating a balloon: The more air you put in the balloon, the bigger it gets, and all of its wrinkles are gone. Higher PEEP can be used for lung inflation especially in the areas of the lungs, which are dependent and have atelectasis. This improves oxygenation.

➤ **Derecruitment:**

This is the process when the pressure is decreased. Like deflation of the balloon, the air gets out quickly, resulting in the complete collapse of the balloon when it shrivels and wrinkles up. Lungs are like balloons; when the PEEP is taken out or decreased, the lung has more areas of atelectasis.

ARDSnet Study:

➤ Tidal volume (TV) 6cc/kg ideal body weight
➤ Plateau pressure Pplat 30-50 cm H2O
➤ Respiratory rate (set ventilatory rate) 6-35 breaths per minute
➤ Weaning by protocol
➤ **FIO2/PEEP combinations:**

0.3/5 0.4/8 0.5/10 0.7/14 0.8/16 0.9/18 1.0/20

Prone Position Ventilation:

➤ **Definition:** This is one of the novel treatment modalities in the management of patients with ARDS. The patients are ventilated in a prone position rather than supine position.

➤ **Pros:** "Proning" improves oxygenation by providing the optimal perfusion to the better ventilated area, therefore improving the ventilation/perfusion (V/Q) ratio.

➤ **Cons:** It is quite cumbersome, especially if done manually. However, there are "proning" beds, which rotate automatically according to a pre-set schedule (rotation occurs every four hours). There may be accidental extubation by dislodgement of the ET tubes or an inadvertent loss of central or arterial lines during the prone position. It is quite challenging to perform procedures such as re-intubation or placing central or arterial lines in these patients. These patients often are on neuromuscular blocking agents, in an induced or artificial coma, and require one-to-one nursing care.

➢ **Consensus statement:** No definite data exist so far, as the jury is still out on the benefit of this treatment modality. It does not reduce the overall mortality from ARDS; however, on the flip side, it does buy you more time so other treatments modalities have a chance to work, i.e., antibiotics kick in for the patient with bacterial pneumonia, while maintaining optimal oxygenation.

Pulmonary Embolism (PE)

➢ **Definition:** Blockage of the blood supply to the lung, caused by a blood clot. The blood clot usually originates in the lower extremity or a pelvic vein (thrombosis). It dislodges from the site of formation, and emigrates to the pulmonary vascular bed (embolism), where it gets embedded in the vascular meshwork.

➢ **DVT** - 50% of DVTs are complicated by PE
   - source of almost all PEs
   - >90% originate from proximal deep veins in the lower extremity
   - **Ilio-femoral vein** is the most common source for PE
   - In women → pelvic veins (a rare but important source)
   - Smoking and birth control pills predispose to DVT/PE

➢ Pathogenesis:
   - Virchow's Triad

➢ **Venous Stasis**
   - Immobility
   - Anesthesia
   - Congestive heart failure

➢ **Hypercoagulable State**
- Factor V leiden deficiency (most common)
- Anti-thrombin III deficiency
- Protein C & S deficiency
- Anticardiolipin antibody
- Nephrotic syndrome
- Malignancy
- Hormonal replacement therapy (estrogen)

➢ **Vessel Wall Injury**
- Trauma
- Surgery

➢ **Clinical signs and symptoms:**
- Leg pain or calf pain (positive Homan's sign in 50% patients with DVT)
- Shortness of breath
- Chest pain
- Cough
- Tachypnea/tachycardia
- Hypoxia
- EKG findings: Usually non-specific ST changes. Massive PE usually present with the right ventricular strain pattern: $\Rightarrow S_1 Q_3 T_3$

➢ **Laboratory:**
- Leukocytosis
- ↑ ESR, ↑ LDH
- ABG: hypoxemia, hypocapnea (low paCO2), respiratory alkalosis
- Troponin I & T are elevated
- Positive d-dimer
  - Lack of specificity, but high sensitivity
  - False positive in:
    - Surgery
    - Trauma
    - Renal disease

- □ Hypercapnia and respiratory acidosis
- □ Pregnancy
- □ Pneumonia
- □ Congestive heart failure (CHF)

➢ **Clinical Presentations:**
- Atelectasis or pulmonary parenchymal abnormalities
- Pleural effusion (47%)
- Most classic findings (not seen in every patient):
  - □ Peripheral wedge-shaped infarct "Hampton's Hump," mostly seen with pulmonary infarct

➢ **Diagnosis:**
- Venography = Old Gold Standard!
- Color flow Doppler (most common)
  - □ Sensitivity = 89%-100%
  - □ Specificity = 89%-100%
- Impedance plethysmography (research purpose)
  - □ High sensitivity
  - □ Low specificity and cost compared to venous ultrasound
- Magnetic resonance venography
  - □ Sensitivity and specificity is equal to venography
  - □ Not operator-dependent
- Pulmonary angiogram
  - □ Confirms or excludes PE with certainty
  - □ Most definitive diagnostic test
  - □ Positive result consists of:
    1. Filling defects
    2. Sharp cut-off of small vessel ("Westermark's Sign")
  - □ Mortality < 0.5%
  - □ Can detect clots as small as 0.5 mm
- Spiral/helical CT chest with contrast
  Sensitivity = 85%
  Specificity = 90%
  Good for proximal pulmonary arteries.
  Low sensitivity for segmental and small, chronic PEs

V/Q RESULTS	OUTCOME & RECOMMENDATIONS
Normal	Excludes PE especially when combined with other diagnostic modality, i.e., negative d-dimer
Low Probability	Further testing may be indicated, especially when the clinical suspicion for a PE is high
Intermediate Probability	
High Probability	PE in the right clinical context, unless proven otherwise

VENTILATION SCAN (Equal ventilation both lungs)

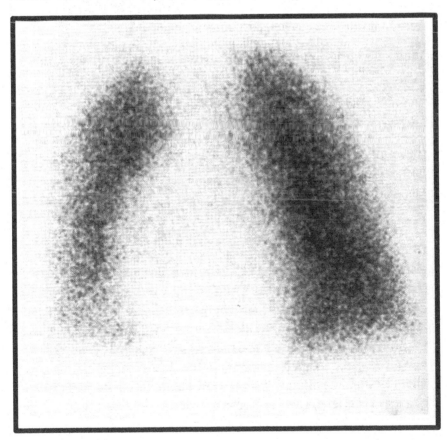

PERFUSION SCAN (no perfusion on the right lung)

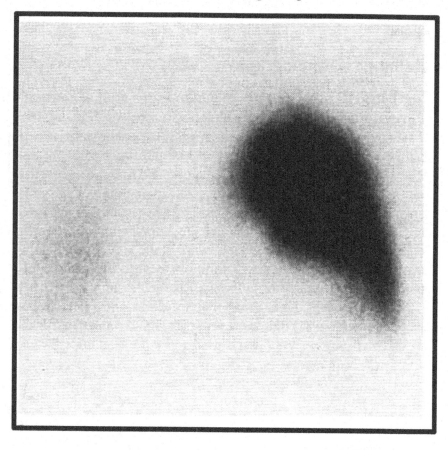

RIGHT PULMONARY ARTERY EMBOLISM (PE)

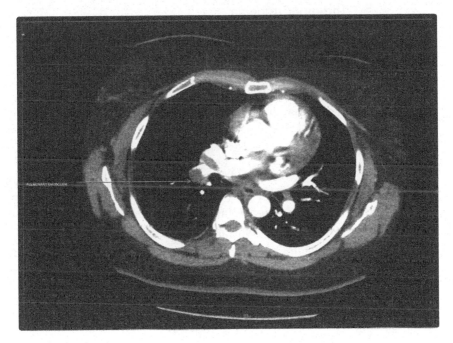

➤ **Treatment:**

- Anticoagulation therapy with heparin (high or low molecular weight) should be initiated at the first clinical suspicion of a PE.
- Dosage is weight dependent, with an initial loading dose of 80 mg of heparin followed by 18 mg/hour and adjusted per the PTT. Meanwhile, LMWH such as Lovenox is started and maintained at 1 mg/kg, divided every 12 hours, given subcutaneously. LMWH usually does not require laboratory monitoring; however, Factor X-a levels can be checked to monitor the anticoagulation effect, especially in patients with breakthrough DVT/PE (patients who develop a new DVT/PE while being on full-dose anticoagulation).
- May require large doses to overcome heparin resistance
- Therapeutic level is at least 1.5-2 times the upper limit of normal PTT range (25-35 seconds)

- Side effects include:
  - Thrombocytopenia
  - Osteoporosis
  - Bleeding is one of the side effects, and when it occurs:
- Stop the heparin infusion
- Give protamine sulfate (antidote)
- Simultaneous initiation of heparin and warfarin is suggested:
  - Effective
  - Shorter hospital stay
- Anticoagulant effect of warfarin is delayed until all clotting factors are cleared from the system, which may take 36-72 hours after warfarin is started. Initially factor VII, with a half-life of 5-7 hours, is cleared. Adequate anticoagulation is not achieved due to the presence of II, IX, and X. In fact, the patient is hypercoagulable and hence requires the overlap with heparin or Lovenox for five days.
- Low molecular weight heparin (LMWH)
  These agents are used for prevention (0.5mg/kg) and treatment of (1 mg/kg) DVT/PE

➢ **Advantages:**
- High bioavailability, longer half-life, less chances of thrombocytopenia, and can be administered subcutaneously.
  Lab monitoring usually is not required; however, Factor X-a can be measured in patients with breakthrough venous thromboembolism or VTE (new clots despite use of appropriate weight-based anticoagulant regimen).

➢ **Thrombolytic therapy:**
Thrombolytic or "clot busters" are used to lyse or break the clot. Most commonly used agent is tPA.
These are useful in life-threatening PE with the following conditions:
- Hemodynamic instability with obstructive shock or respiratory compromise, requiring vasopressors and

mechanical ventilation
- PE with a new onset of right-sided heart failure
➤ Percutaneous Mechanical Thrombectomy:
  - It is a procedure performed through the internal jugular or subclavian venous access for the clot fragmentation and aspiration
➤ **Indications:**
  - Massive PE (Saddle PE)
  - Right ventricular failure
➤ **Contraindications to Tissue Thromboplastin (TPA):**
  - High bleeding risk or active bleeding
  - Surgical thrombectomy is unavailable
➤ **Indications for Intravenous Filters (IVC Filters):**
Acute DVT when conventional anticoagulation is contraindicated:
  - Recent surgery
  - Hemorrhagic stroke
  - Active bleeding
  - Acute venous thromboembolism in which anticoagulant has been ineffective
  - Pulmonary vascular bed is significantly compromised, e.g.,
    - Massive PE with huge pulmonary clot burden
    - Chronic recurrent and unprovoked thromboembolism
➤ **Complications of IVC Filters:**
Overall mortality from placement of an IVC filter remains very low:
  - Complications due to insertion process (bleeding, infection)
  - Venous thrombosis at the insertion site
  - Filter migration
  - Filter erosion through the IVC wall
  - IVC obstruction
  - Pulmonary hypertension

Sepsis Syndrome

> ➤ **Definition:**

It is a constellation of clinical symptoms, which are caused by a variety of insults ranging from infection (pneumonia, UTI) to noninfectious causes such as trauma. Clinical presentation ranges from SIRS to septic shock. Typically it is an exaggerated and unchecked inflammatory response to certain stimuli, i.e., infection, trauma, pancreatitis.

- **Systemic Inflammatory Response Syndrome (SIRS):**
Generalized inflammatory response to infection or noninfectious causes, leading to harmful and unregulated host immune response

> ➤ **Clinical Manifestation of SIRS:**

- Core temperature > 38° C or < 36° C
- Tachycardia (>90 beats/min)
- Tachypnea (>20 breaths/min, $PaCO_2$ <32 mm Hg, or requirement of mechanical ventilation)
- White blood cell count >12 000/mm3 or <4 000 mm 3 or >10% mature neutrophils
- Can lead to septic shock, multi-organ failure, and death

> ➤ **Sepsis Cascade:**

- SIRS
- Sepsis
- Severe sepsis
- Septic shock
- Severe shock with multi-organ failure

> ➤ **Septic Shock:**

It is characterized by low blood pressure, disseminated intravascular coagulation (DIC), metabolic disturbances, and multiple organ failure

> ➤ **Clinical manifestations:**

- **Hyperdynamic shock**
  - This type of septic shock typically occurs during the initial phase of sepsis.

- It is characterized by an increased cardiac output and the loss of peripheral resistance.
- Occurs due to massive vasodilation and vascular leak caused by the release of pro-inflammatory cytokines (TNF-α and IL-1β), nitric oxide, and prostaglandins
- Caused by an inadequate supply of metabolic substrate (oxygen), resulting in anaerobic glycolysis and leading to lactic acidosis and tissue damage (Krebs's cycle). Lactate level usually is greater than two.
- ScvO2 (mixed venous oxygen saturations) is less than 70 (range 70 to 90)

- **Respiratory Failure**
  - Results due to extreme demands on lungs at times when airway resistance and capillary leak are increased
  - Respiratory system compliance decreases, hence muscle efficiency is impaired
  - Approximately 85% of septic patients require mechanical ventilatory support (BIPAP, ventilator) or supplemental oxygen

- **Multiple Organ Failure**
  - Caused by tissue hypoperfusion and hypoxia
  - Ultimate cause of death in patients with septic shock

- **Disseminated Intravascular Coagulation (DIC)**
  - Characterized by widespread microvascular thrombosis and profuse bleeding
  - Thrombosis is due to the deposition of fibrin, which results in the occlusion of capillaries, impairing forward blood flow.
  - Bleeding is caused by depletion of the coagulation proteins and platelets from continued and uncontrolled activation of the coagulation system.
  - Xigris is a recombinant-activated protein-C that replaces the protein-C-deficient milieu in septic shock.

It prevents the formation of the microthrombi in the vasculature. It has been taken off the market, due to the lack of clear benefits and side effects such as bleeding. It is still available for use on compassionate grounds.

➢ **Signs and symptoms:**

- Infection is coupled with tachycardia, tachypnea, and shortness of breath
- Lactic acidosis buildup due to anaerobic glycolysis
- Altered state of consciousness, which may present as confusion, agitation, anxiety, or psychosis. A combination of hypoxemia and hypotension leads to impaired cerebral blood flow and confusion
- Reduced urinary output and abnormal bilirubin levels due to reduced kidney function ("shocked kidney"), and diminished liver function ("shocked liver"). This reflects impaired organ perfusion due to both hypotension and microthrombi depleting flow to the visceral microvasculature.
- Red skin lesions (mottling or purpuric lesions)
- *Purpura fulminans*: Acute onset of cutaneous hemorrhage and necrosis in 25% patient's population with meningococcemia (septicemia caused by Neisseria meningitidis). This usually involves trunk and lower extremities. Thrombocytopenia and DIC is the underlying cause of the purpuric lesions seen in *purpura fulminans*.

➢ **Laboratory Biomarkers:**

- **C-reactive protein (CRP)** is an acute-phase reactant which is a protein-based enzyme released by the liver after onset of inflammation or as a result of tissue damage. It is a commonly used marker to differentiate between viral/bacterial infections and inflammation (nonspecific marker). However, it is elevated during any stress, infection, or inflammation.

- **Procalcitonin** is a more valuable marker for the diagnosis of sepsis. Its concentration highly correlates with the severity of the disease.

➢ **Treatment:**

- Treatment regimen includes institution of an appropriate empiric antibiotic regimen, removal of the source of infection (if known) through wound debridement, and removal of infected hardware. It also entails providing hemodynamic, respiratory, and metabolic support while other treatment modalities are used.

- The concept of early goal-directed therapy (EGDT) is applied once sepsis is identified, often in the ER setting. Aggressive fluid resuscitation should be given to the patients when the serum lactate levels are >4. This should be followed by placement of a central line in the IJ or subclavian vein to monitor CVP (ideal CVP numbers are 8-10). The central venous access should have the capability to monitor the ScvO2 continuously. The goal is to keep the ScvO2 between 70-90; if less than 70, and the CVP>8, then add dobutamine to increase the cardiac output in order to maintain organ perfusion.

- Vasopressor therapy using intravenous administration of norepinephrine or dopamine. Vasopressors, often referred to as "pressors," increase peripheral vascular constriction, thus enhancing venous return to the heart and help with the tissue perfusion.

- Ventilatory support using BIPAP or conventional ventilators

- Insulin therapy is required to maintain blood glucose levels between 100-150 mg/dl, which helps improve neutrophil mediated phagocytosis.

- Hydrocortisone, in physiological doses of 100 mg IV every eight hours, is recommended in patients with septic shock who are often on vasopressors for the hemodynamic support. A random serum cortisol level is recommended in a septic patient at baseline to screen for the adrenal insufficiency. Cortisol level of less than 25 mg/dl in a hemodynamically unstable patient is suggestive of a relative adrenal insufficiency.

➢ **Complications:**
- Acute respiratory distress syndrome (ARDS)
- Disseminated intravascular coagulation (DIC)
- Acute renal failure (ARF)
- Intestinal bleeding
- Liver failure
- Central nervous system dysfunction
- Heart failure

Toxic Shock Syndrome (TSS)

➢ **Definition:**

A potentially fatal clinical syndrome characterized by symptoms of shock, caused by release of the bacterial toxins. The symptom onset is quite sudden. The most common culprit is *Staphylococcus* bacteria, commonly referred to as "Staph." Streptococcus bacteria Group A-streptococcus on the other hand is also toxic shock-like syndrome (TSLS).

➢ **Pathophysiology:**

It is a toxin-mediated exotoxin process, when toxins are released in response to the underlying infection. The most common are TSS toxin type-1(TSST-1) and staphylococcal enterotoxin-B. The majority of patients have developed antibodies to these toxins by adolescence. Patients who fail to develop this antibody response are predisposed to develop the deleterious effects of toxic shock. The toxins are absorbed systemically, and in susceptible patients these toxins will form super-antigens. These super-antigens, in turn, will work on T-cells and cytokines, causing an exaggerated inflammatory mediated response. This results in the clinical sequalae of TSS.

➤ **Epidemiology:**
The incidence of TSS historically has been more common amongst females due to tampon use. However, the incidence has been declining precipitously due to unavailability of the highly absorbent tampons. It is more common in the Western Hemisphere.

➤ **Sign and Symptoms:**
- SIRS/sepsis
- Rash
- Septic shock
- Hemodynamic/circulatory failure
- Renal failure
- ARDS, secondary to the capillary leak
- Coagulopathy

➤ **Diagnosis:**
- Based on clinical grounds, i.e., new infection, rash, especially in susceptible patients
- No single lab test is confirmatory for the diagnosis
- Pan-culture is usually recommended, prior to the empiric antibiotic

➤ **Treatment:**
- Intensive care monitoring is required
- Hemodynamic support, IV fluids, or vasopressors, as needed
- Removal of the source of infection, tampons, nasal package, barrier contraceptives, or surgical dressings
- Incision and drainage of the infected wound or abscess
- Empiric antibiotic regimen tailored to cover for the suspected pathogens
- Supportive care including respiratory support, i.e., supplemental oxygen, invasive or noninvasive ventilation as needed
- Hemodialysis if renal failure
- Intravenous immune globulins (IVIG) may be indicated in severe cases

Lemierre's Disease (LD)

➤ **Definition:**

It is showering of the septic emboli to the lung and other major organs. The infection originates in the vicinity of the neck soft tissue vasculature. The jugular vein is often the source of septic emboli. The infection could originate from a infected tooth or a peritonsillar abscess.

History: First reported by Dr. Andre Lemierre in 1936. It was initially termed as "post-anginal septicemia."

Microorganisms: Fusobacterium necrophorum, from the tonsillar and peritonsillar area, is the most common source of infection. It is not a contagious infection, since it emanates from the disruption of normal oral/dental flora as a result of local trauma or infection.

➤ **Symptoms:**
- Sore throat
- Lethargy
- Fever and malaise
- Shortness of breath
- Chest pain
- Pneumonia
- Tenderness in the front and side of the neck
- Swollen lymph nodes in the neck area
- Joint pain

➤ **Diagnosis:**
- CT/MRI of the chest, head, and neck
- Blood culture
- TEE (transesophageal echocardiogram)

➤ **Treatment:**

Antibiotics covering gram positive, gram negative, and anaerobes should be used as the infection can be poly-microbial. Six weeks or a longer treatment may be necessary to successfully treat the infection and the associated septic emboli.

DVT prophylaxis with heparin or LMWH is usually recommended.

Lemierre's Disease (multiple septic emboli)

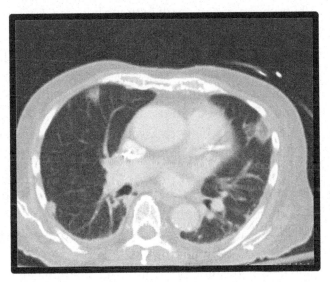

Hypoxia

> **Definition:**
> It is a state of relative oxygen deficiency, which is character-
> ized by organ dysfunction such as mental confusion, chest
> pain, or shortness of breath. Sometimes hypoxia may manifest
> as MI, stroke, or respiratory failure.

> **Types of Hypoxia:**
> - **Hypoxic Hypoxia:** It is described as a lack of oxygen con-
>   centration. It tends to occur at high altitudes when the air
>   is "thin," or with the use of faulty oxygen equipment (hos-
>   pital setting, patient transport, or in high-altitude aircraft
>   and during high-altitude climbs).
> - **Hypemic Hypoxia:** Cigarette smoking or use of certain
>   medications can cause an increased carbon monox-
>   ide concentration in the blood. It reduces the enzymes
>   needed for the oxygen transport, therefore rendering a
>   relatively hypoxic state.
> - **Stagnant Hypoxia:** Restricted circulation, i.e., application

of tourniquets, or exposure to extreme cold temperatures (hypothermia) can result in tissue hypoxia. G-forces (gravitational forces) affect blood circulation during high-speed maneuvering in military aircrafts. These maneuvers can also deprive the vital organs of oxygen supply by pooling the blood in the dependent body parts, i.e., lower extremity. This results in tissue hypoperfusion and hypoxia, typically called Gravity-associated Loss of Consciousness (G-LOC), especially in military aircrafts, which can result in an aviation mishap.

- **Histotoxic Hypoxia:** Hypoxia caused by damaging effects of certain medications, such as metformin and HIV/AIDS medications. These medications cause mitochondrial dysfunction, thus impairing the aerobic glycolysis. Smoke inhalation, cyanide poisoning, and alcohol can have similar toxic effects.

➢ **Symptoms of Hypoxia:**

There are a variety of hypoxic symptoms that are pertinent to the organ involved. These symptoms could be confusion, apprehension, fatigue, headache, belligerence, numbness, tingling, blurred vision, hot/cold flushes, and occasionally euphoria, especially when CNS is involved. Patient may experience chest pain or shortness of breath when heart or lungs are affected.

➢ **Sign of Hypoxia:**

Hyperventilation, cyanosis, mental confusion, poor judgment, ataxia, poor muscle coordination

➢ **Treatment of Hypoxia:**
- First provide oxygen as soon as possible
- "Find and fix" the underlying cause of hypoxia

Decompression Sickness (DCS) "Bends"

➢ **Definition:**

A clinical syndrome characterized by a myriad of symptoms due to a decrease in the ambient pressure resulting in the formation of nitrogen bubbles in the circulation. These bubbles form in the bloodstream and other organ systems. The bubbles not only impair the perfusion but also result in direct tissue damage due to the osmotic pressure.

➤ **Pathophysiology:**

The body is composed of a mixture of gasses. It is 79% nitrogen and 21% oxygen. Various gas laws affect the physical and chemical properties of these gases, i.e., especially when subjected to extreme atmospheric pressures changes both under water and at higher altitude. This phenomenon of DCS is observed more often in underwater divers when they return to the surface too quickly after their dive. Severity of symptoms is directly correlated with length and depth of the dive. Similar phenomenon occurs at higher altitudes, when the body is subjected to a very low barometric pressure.

➤ **Clinical Manifestation:**

- **Type I:** *"Grecian bends"* are cutaneous manifestations of DCS with no serious sequalae. The clinical presentation of the bends may include:
  - Pruritus
  - Rash (cutaneous marmorata)
  - Lymphatic obstruction
- **Type II:** *"Chokers or Staggers"* respiratory or systemic manifestations
  - Musculoskeletal (joint or muscle pain)
  - 30% may progress to systemic manifestations
  - "Chokes" (pertaining to "choking") are pulmonary manifestation of the DCS, characterized by chest pain, dyspnea, or cough. CXR may show pulmonary edema.
  - "Staggers" (pertaining to ataxia, balance, or gait disturbances) is the neurological manifestation of the DCS, and results in ataxia and lack of coordination, hence the term "staggers."

- **Type III:** Catastrophic/Fatal manifestations
- Most severe form of DCS, which results in multi-organ failure and death

➤ **Risk Factors that predispose to DCS:**
- Lack of knowledge and necessary training prior to the dive or exposure to extreme altitudes
- Gender F>M
- Age >40 years
- Dehydration
- Alcohol use

➤ **Diagnosis:**
- Clinical history suggesting either diving or high-altitude flying immediately prior to the symptoms onset
- Blood pressure cuff test: The test is considered positive when inflating the BP cuff around the affected joint and muscle group relieves the symptoms of DCS, i.e., pain and paresthesia

➤ **Treatment:**
- Hyperbaric chamber therapy
- 100% oxygen during high altitudes and descend whenever possible
- Immobilize the affected area

Critical Care Cardiology

1. **Hemodynamic Support**
   a) Vasopressors and Inotropes
   b) Intra-Aortic Balloon Pumps (IABP)
2. **Acute Coronary Syndromes**
   a) NSTEMI
   b) STEMI
3. **Acute CHF Management**
4. **High Output Cardiac Failure**
5. **Heart Failure Classification**
6. **Pulmonary Hypertension**
7. **Multi-Focal Atrial Tachycardia (MAT)**
8. **Cardiac Resynchronization Therapy (CRT)**
9. **Pulseless Electrical Activity (PEA)**
10. **Systemic Vascular Resistance (SVR)**
11. **Ventricular Assist Device (VAD) or "Heart Pump"**
12. **Supra-Ventricular Tachycardia (SVT)**
13. **Atrial Fibrillation/Atrial Flutter (A-Fib/A-Flutter)**
14. **Cardiac Tamponade**
15. **Acute Aortic Dissection**
16. **Hypertensive Urgency**
17. **Hypertensive Emergency**
18. **Malignant Hypertension**

Hemodynamic Support

INOTROPES AND VASOPRESSORS

➤ **Dopamine:**
- It is a vasopressor that works on various receptors depending on the dose, resulting in a myriad of responses:
  - **Low Dose (<5):** works on the dopamine receptors at lower doses and cause vasodilation of the renal vessels (previously referred to as *renal-dose-dopa*). No longer used for renal perfusion
  - **Moderate Dose (5-10):** Causes beta-1 stimulation, resulting in tachycardia and increase in blood pressure
  - **Higher Doses (>10):** Causes more alpha-1 activity. It offers less benefits in patient with septic shock, who often have preexisting tachycardia

➤ **Epinephrine:**
- It primarily is used as the first agent in every ACLS scenario with cardiac arrest. "God's Drug" since it has shown to help during the code situations
  - Beta-1 and beta-2 activity along with the alpha-1 (vasoconstrictor properties)
  - May decrease splanchnic blood flow

➤ **Norepinephrine (Levophed):**
- It has more alpha than beta properties
  - Drug of choice in septic shock
  - Causes less tachycardia
  - Improves tissue perfusion

➤ **Phenylephrine:**
- It causes profound arterial vasoconstriction
  - Good as an anesthetic reversal agent
  - Works on the alpha receptors

➤ **Vasopressin:**
- It causes vasoconstriction by working on the V-1-receptors
  - Better side effect profile than norepinephrine in

patients with mild septic shock

- ◻ Normally, vasopressin concentrations are increased as a response to hypotension. This normal physiologic response is blunted in patients with septic shock. Infusing vasopressin in patients with septicemia reflect replacement of vasopressin, which has been suppressed as a result of sepsis
- ◻ May caused cardiac ischemia in susceptible individuals

➤ **Isoproterenol:**
- ▪ Works as an chronotropic agent on beta-1 and beta 2 receptors
  - ◻ It can be used in symptomatic bradycardia
  - ◻ May provoke cardiac arrhythmias

➤ **Dobutamine:**
- ▪ It is an Inotropic agent
  - ◻ Used in low cardiac output scenarios
  - ◻ Unpredictable blood pressure response
  - ◻ Not a vasopressor agent

➤ **Milrinone:**
- ▪ It is a phosphodiesterase inhibitor (PDE)
  - ◻ Works by vasodilation
  - ◻ Decreases pre-load and pulmonary arterial pressures
  - ◻ May cause coagulopathy
  - ◻ Increases mortality in patients with heart failure
    - – Alpha receptors have vasoconstrictor properties that enhance venous return
    - – Beta receptors have cardiac properties, i.e., increase heart rate

Intra-Aortic Balloon Pump (IABP)

- ▪ Placed percutaneously, usually through the femoral artery. The balloon tip ends distal to the left subclavian artery
- ▪ Works on the principles of counter-pulsation. Its pulsation

during diastole helps perfuse the heart and deflation during systole creates a negative force drawing the blood flow in the forward direction.

- Benefits of decreased after-load are more convincingly demonstrated than coronary perfusion
- Can be set at 1:1, 1:2, or 1:3 (Inflations: Heart Beats Ratio) 1:3 is a weaning modality
- Critical to maintain anticoagulation as clots can form while being on the pump
- Complications
  □ Mesenteric ischemia
  □ Lower extremity ischemia
  □ Helium embolization
  □ Balloon rupture

Acute Coronary Syndromes
➢ **Pathophysiology:**
- Imbalance between oxygen supply and demand
- Myocardial ischemia
- Coronary perfusion decreases due to stenosis, vasospasm, or a thrombus

➢ **Treatment:**
- Use the acronym **MONA**:
  □ **M**orphine – helps with the pain control only. The benefits of decreased O2 demand has no impact on morbidity/mortality
  □ **O**xygen – enhances supply of oxygen
  □ **N**itroglycerin – venodilatory effects
  □ **A**spirin – improves survival by preventing platelet aggregation
- Beta blocker – Decrease myocardial oxygen demand by slowing the heart rate
- Anti-platelet agents, i.e., clopidogrel (Plavix) or prasugrel, adds to the anti-platelet properties of aspirin

- Anticoagulation with heparin and Lovenox (for NSTEMI) to prevent clot propagation
- Cardiac catheterization with angioplasty and/or stenting (for STEMI) to reopen occluded vessels
- Revascularization: CABG if triple vessel or left main disease

NON-ST SEGMENT ELEVATION MYOCARDIAL INFARCTION (NSTEMI)

- ➤ **Definition:** Myocardial infarction without EKG evidence of ST segment elevation (troponins are elevated)
- ➤ **Treatment:**
  - Morphine (pain control, no mortality benefit)
  - Oxygen to meet the increased oxygen demand
  - Nitrates provide venodilatory effects, however offer no mortality benefit
  - Aspirin 325 mg
  - Anticoagulant (heparin or low molecular weight heparin)
  - Clopidogrel (Plavix)
    - 20% reduction in CV death, MI, and CVA
    - Relatively contraindicated if CABG anticipated or planed within the next few days
- ➤ **Percutaneous Coronary Intervention:**
  - Relatively contraindicated in low-risk patients
  - Must occur within 48-96 hours of presentation
  - A IIB/IIIA receptor antagonist should be used if coronary intervention is contemplated

ST-ELEVATION MI (STEMI)

- ➤ Initial contact with paramedics system to the catheterization lab time should be <30 minutes.
- ➤ Angioplasty should be performed within 90 minutes of arrival to the hospital (door to needle time should be less than 90 minutes).
- ➤ Initial management is otherwise identical to NSTEMI.

> ➤ Hospitals should have an expedited transfer protocol in place if a 24/7 in-house catheterization lab is not available.
> ➤ Management of myocardial infarction is one of the core measures set forth by the CMS to evaluate and grade hospitals and cardiac catheterization labs.

Acute CHF Management

➤ **Aldosterone Antagonist, Spironolactone:**
  - Decreases mortality by 24% in NYHC III-IV
  - Mode of action
    - Mild diuretic
    - Ventricular remodeling
  - Side effect
    - Hyperkalemia, especially with ACE-I/ARB combination; therefore, close monitoring of the potassium level is required

➤ **Eplerenone:**
  - Similar to spironolactone
  - Decreased mortality by 42% in NYHC III-IV with EF<35

➤ **Diuretics:**
  - Loop diuretic, furosemide (Lasix), bumetanide (Bumex)
  - No impact on mortality
  - Reduces the pre-load; however, electrolyte monitoring is required as hyponatremia and hypokalemia can result.
  - Over-diuresis can result in contraction alkalosis

➤ **Brain Natriuretic Peptide (BNP) Nesiritide:**
  - Arterial and venous vasodilation
  - Natriuresis/diuresis
  - May be associated with renal insufficiency
  - Increases mortality, therefore no longer used in the critical care setting

➤ **Digitalis Compounds, Digoxin:**
  - Decreases hospitalizations
  - No impact on mortality

- Requires monitoring of levels as digoxin has a narrow therapeutic index
➤ **Inotropic Agent, Dobutamine:**
  - Increases mortality; therefore, cautious and judicious use is indicated
➤ *Beta-blockers are relatively contraindicated in acute, decompensated CHF. However, if the patient has been on stable doses of beta blockers, these can be continued safely on the same doses*

High Output Heart Failure

➤ **Definition:** Signs and symptoms of congestive heart failure (CHF) with high cardiac output status. Cardiac Index (CI >4 L/M/M2)
➤ **Etiology:**
  - Multiple myeloma - 23%
    - Due to hyper-vascularity and AV shunting, similar to Paget's disease
  - Hyperthyroidism
  - Beriberi (vitamin B1 deficiency)
  - Arteriovenous (AV) malformation, which is surgically created for hemodialysis. It can occasionally occur as a complication of a stab or gunshot wound, which may result in a pathologic arteriovenous anastomosis.
  - Paget's disease, which causes hyper-vascularity within the bone marrow and shunting of the blood across the vessels
➤ **Clinical:**
  - Symptoms of CHF, chest pain, shortness of breath, generalized swelling
  - Increased pulmonary capillary wedge pressure (PCWP), which is simply referred to as a wedge pressure >18 mm Hg
  - Decreased pulmonary vascular resistance (PVR)
➤ **Diagnosis:**
  - Quantitative scan

- □ Increased radioactivity in the bones
- □ Increased radioactivity in lungs with a left to right shunt

Heart Failure Classification
New York Heart Association (NYHA) Classification
I   No symptoms with ordinary physical activity (asymptomatic)
II   Symptoms with ordinary activities but only slight limitation of activities (minimal symptoms on maximal exercise)
III Marked physical limitations symptoms with minimal activity (maximal symptoms at minimal exercise)
IV   Symptoms with any activity or even at rest (symptomatic at rest)

Pulmonary Hypertension
- ➤ **Diagnosis:** Clinical condition characterized by a mean arterial pressure (MAP) over 25 mmHg at rest, and >30 with exercise. It should ideally be measured by placing the Swan-Ganz catheter (SGC). Right ventricular systolic pressure (RVSP) >40 estimated by an echocardiogram can be used as a surrogate marker for the elevated pulmonary pressures. The RVSP is measured by calculating the tricuspid regurgitant velocity on echocardiogram.
- ➤ **WHO Classification:**
  - ▪ **Group I** Pulmonary arterial hypertension—idiopathic, familial
    Congenital heart/valvular diseases (CVD), connective tissue diseases, i.e., scleroderma
    Porto-pulmonary hypertension (cirrhosis)
    HIV/AIDS
    Diet medications such as fen-phen
  - ▪ **Group II** Acquired left heart disease, valvular, or ischemic heart disease
  - ▪ **Group III** Lung disease/hypoxemia
    - □ OSA, COPD, IPF

- **Group IV** Chronic thromboembolic pulmonary hypertension (CTEPH); Venous thromboembolic disease (VTE), i.e., PE
- **Group V** Miscellaneous, i.e., sarcoidosis, fibrosing mediastinitis

➢ **Severity Index:**

Graded by the functional classification

➢ **Work-up needed for the diagnosis of pulmonary hypertension:**
  - ANA (connective tissue disease screen)
  - PFT (to assess underlying lung function for the determination of the COPD, ILD, or other lung conditions causing hypoxia)
  - Sleep study (polysomnography-PSG) to rule out sleep related breathing disorders
  - Right heart catheterization by Swan-Ganz catheter placement
  - Ventilation-perfusion scan (V/Q scan) to check for chronic small PEs
  - Liver function tests (LFTs), hepatitis serology, and HIV testing may be indicated in selected patient population

Multi-focal Atrial Tachycardia (MAT)

➢ **Definition:**
  - Irregular, narrow complex tachycardia with three or more distinct P wave morphologies on the EKG or rhythm strips
  - Automatic arrhythmia associated with severe respiratory disease (COPD), cardiac drugs, theophylline, and any pulmonary pathology such as an acute PE or pneumonia

➢ **Treatment:**
  - Eliminate predisposing factors:
    - Discontinue theophylline
    - Reverse hypoxemia
    - Treat lactic acidosis
    - Optimize CHF/respiratory status

- Amiodarone
- Calcium channel blocker
➢ **Contraindicated:**
  - Beta blockers—worsen bronchospasm during acute COPD/asthma exacerbation
  - Electric cardio-version
  - Digoxin

Cardiac Resynchronization Therapy (CRT)
➢ **Definition:**

Placement of biventricular pacing in CHF Class III or IV (with asynchrony-LBBB)

MIRACLE TRIAL
- Improved LV contractility
- Decreased mortality
- Improved symptoms at six months

COMPANION TRIAL
- CRT +/- defibrillator improves survival as compared with the medical treatment alone

DIG TRIAL
- Digoxin is usually not helpful as the levels <1 are preferable

➢ **Medical Treatment:**
  - ACE-I
  - Beta blocker
  - Spironolactone
  - Digoxin

Pulseless Electrical Activity (PEA)
➢ **Look for, and treat the underlying etiology (5 Hs, and 5 Ts):**
➢ **H (5):**
  - Hypovolemia
  - Hypoxia
  - Hydrogen ion (acidosis)

- Hypo/hyperkalemia or electrolyte imbalances
- Hypothermia
➢ **T (5):**
  - Tamponade, i.e., cardiac tamponade
  - Tablets; medication induced
  - Tension pneumothorax
  - Thrombus (MI)
  - Thromboembolic diseases (PE)

Systemic Vascular Resistance (SVR)
➢ **Systemic Vascular Resistance (SVR):**
  - Mean arterial pressure minus right atrial pressure times eighty divided by cardiac output (MAP-RAPX80/CO)
  - 80 is a constant that converts mmHg to dynes*sec/cm2
  - Normal=770-1600 dynes*sec/cm2
➢ **Systemic Vascular Resistance Index (SVRI):**
  - MAP-RAP*80/CI
  - CI=CO/BSA
  - Normal is 200-2400
➢ **Low to Low Normal SVR:**
  - Early septic shock
  - Neurogenic shock
➢ **High to High Normal SVR:**
  - Late septic shock
  - Hypovolemic shock
  - Obstructive shock
  - Cardiogenic shock

Ventricular Assist Device (VAD) or "Heart Pump"
➢ **Definition:**
  It is a mechanical pump placed in patients with severe cardiomyopathy. It functions to supply the blood to other organs because of intrinsic heart failure. It is often placed as a bridge in patients with cardiomyopathy who are awaiting heart transplant.

➢ **Types:**
  ▪ Left ventricular assist device (LVAD) most common
  ▪ Right ventricular assist device (RVAD)
  ▪ Biventricular assist device (BIVAD)
➢ **Design:**
  ▪ Transcutaneous (short-term)
  ▪ Implantable (long-term)
➢ **Medication/Precautions post implantation:**
  ▪ Coumadin
  ▪ Prevention of infection
  ▪ Learning of the device, alarms, malfunction, and troubleshooting
➢ **Complications post implantation:**
  ▪ Thrombosis
  ▪ Tamponade
  ▪ Arrhythmia
  ▪ Ischemia
  ▪ Hypovolemia
  ▪ Device malfunction
➢ **Cardiac arrest after the implantation:**
  ▪ Standard ACLS protocol, i.e., CPR rules don't apply in this setting
  ▪ Normally there is no pulse or BP by auscultations in patients post implantation due to the continuous blood flow, rather than the normal pulsatile flow. Therefore can't rely on pulse and BP monitoring to assess the hemodynamic status
  ▪ Doppler are used to monitor the BP, and a pressure of 60-90 mmHg is considered normal
  ▪ Pulse oximetery may not be reliable in these patients as well, due to erratic blood flow to the extremities; therefore, ABG is recommended
  ▪ Use patient's mental status, skin turgor to assess the tissue/organ perfusion

- Listen for the continuous "hum" on the left lower rib margin
- In case of thrombosis, TPA can be administered
- Hemodynamic support

Biventricular Ventricular Assist Device (VAD)

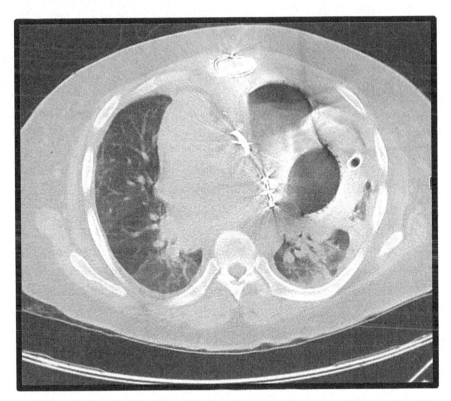

Supra-ventricular Tachycardia

➤ **Definition:** Arrhythmias originating from any anatomical site above the ventricles. These arrhythmias are often characterized by rapid heart rates greater than 100 beats per minute
➤ **Classification (Anatomical):**
- Atrial fibrillation
- Atrial flutter

- Ventricular nodal re-entrant tachycardia (VNRT)
- Ventricular re-entrant tachycardia (VRT)
- Paroxysmal supra-ventricular tachycardia (PSVT)

➢ **Classification (Hemodynamics):**
- **Stable:** Blood pressure is usually stable and patient may be relatively asymptomatic
- **Unstable:** Shock, hemodynamic instability, chest pain, shortness of breath, altered level of consciousness may ensue due to the lack of tissue perfusion

➢ **Pathophysiology:**
Majority of these arrhythmias emanate from an anatomical site located above the ventricles. A host of triggers may be involved in triggering these arrhythmias, such as PE, MI, or other pathologies, which lead to stress on the pulmonary vasculature. The re-entrant tachycardia are caused by an abnormal circulatory loop, which is formed between the atria and ventricles.

➢ **Treatment:**
Management should be directed towards the cause of individual SVTs. As a general principle, if the patient is hemodynamically unstable and symptomatic, an aggressive treatment approach should be used such as electrical or chemical cardioversion. Meanwhile, supportive care should be provided to the patient, such as supplemental oxygen, pain control, and hemodynamic support.

Atrial Fibrillation & Atrial Flutter (A-Fib & A-Flutter)

➢ **Definition:** Arrhythmia originating from the atria or the pulmonary vasculature.

➢ **Classification:**
- **New Onset:** Newly diagnosed, could be either symptomatic or asymptomatic
- **Chronic:** Known, often already diagnosed and/or treated
- **Lone:** One-time incidence of A-fibrillation. This usually

occurs due to any physiological stress, such as PE, MI, etc., and doesn't require prolonged treatment with antiarrhythmic or anticoagulation

- **Paroxysmal:** These are intermittent and episodic arrhythmic events
- **According to the Rate:** When the atrial fibrillation rate is greater than 100 per minute, it is designated as A-fib with Rapid Ventricular Response (RVR). Atrial flutter, on the other hand, presents as variable blocks on the EKG.

➢ **Treatment:**
- Treatment regimen is directed towards the underlying causes. Sometimes it could be a simple fix, such as relieving the pain, replacing electrolytes, and providing fever control. Sometimes complex disease such as PE may be responsible for SVT. These complex etiologies entail an aggressive diagnostic and treatment approach.
- If the symptoms are present for less than 48 hours, then rhythm can be converted to normal sinus rhythm by electrical cardioversion. Generally, anticoagulation is not needed if the timing of the symptoms onset is reliable. However, if the symptoms are prolonged and the onset is unknown, then patient should be anticoagulated prior to the cardioversion. If urgent cardioversion is considered or anticipated and the onset of symptomology is not known, then a TEE should be performed to assess for any thrombus in the heart. This thrombus could potentially dislodge, causing a thromboembolic stroke if a thrombus is not excluded prior to the cardioversion.
- Patients with chronic atrial fibrillation should be evaluated and considered for lifelong anticoagulation, if there are no absolute contraindications to full dose anticoagulation. Risk versus benefit should be weighed before initiation and the throughout the anticoagulation period.

Cardiac Tamponade

> **Definition:** A condition that is characterized by abnormal accumulation of fluid in the pericardial sac. This could be secondary to the serous fluid or blood depending on the underlying etiology.

> **Etiology:**
  - Trauma
  - Post MI
  - Malignancy
  - Infections, TB
  - Collagen vascular disease RA, SLE
  - Sarcoidosis

> **Clinical (Beck's Triad):**
  - Hypotension
  - Jugular venous distension (JVD)
  - Muffled heart sounds

> **Complications:**
  - Hemodynamic collapse
  - Arrhythmia
  - Pulseless electrical activity (PEA)

> **Treatment:**
  - Pericardiocentesis: The fluid may be drained on as needed basis or sometimes continuous pericardial drainage may be required to relieve the tamponade
  - Hemodynamic support, such as fluid and /or vasopressors
  - Respiratory support, if needed

Acute Aortic Dissection

> **Definition:**
  Formation of a false lumen between the tunica intima and media of the aorta, which is caused by the shearing forces

> **Etiology:**
  Trauma
  Prolonged and uncontrolled hypertension

Congenital condition, i.e., Marfan syndrome, Ehler-Danlos syndrome

➢ **Classification (Anatomical Location):**
  ▪ Thoracic
  ▪ Abdominal

➢ **Classification (Thoracic):**
  Stanford:
  ▪ Type A: ascending aorta (requires surgery)
  ▪ Type B: descending aorta (medical management under most cases)
  DeBakey:
  ▪ Type I: Ascending aorta, aortic arch, and descending aorta
  ▪ Type II: Ascending aorta
  ▪ Type II: Descending aorta distal to the left subclavian artery

➢ **Treatment:**
  Surgery is the treatment of choice, depending on the location, chronicity, nature, and rate of progression rather than the aneurysm size. However, once the diameter increases to greater than 8-10, a surgical evaluation is needed.

  Supportive measure such as blood pressure (Target SBP<110) and optimal pain control

Hypertensive Urgency

➢ **Definition:**
  Hypertensive urgency is a severe elevation in blood pressure without progressive end-organ dysfunction, i.e., no evidence of renal failure, CAD, or mental confusion. Hypertensive urgency is a situation in which blood pressure should be lowered within a few hours.

➢ **Diagnosis:**
  The distinction between emergencies and urgencies is important because it often dictates the treatment modality

appropriate for the management. Patients with target-organ damage, such as encephalopathy or aortic dissection, require emergent blood-pressure reduction with intensive monitoring and parenteral drug therapy. A fundoscopic examination is particularly useful because it can distinguish a true hypertensive emergency from hypertensive urgency (the presence of new hemorrhages, exudates, or papilledema indicates emergency).

➤ **Etiology:**
- Essential hypertension
- Renovascular disease
  - Acute glomerulonephritis
  - Vasculitis
  - Hemolytic uremic syndrome (HUS)
  - Thrombotic thrombocytopenic purpura (TTP)
  - Renal artery stenosis (RAS)
- Pregnancy
  - Eclampsia
- Endocrine
  - Pheochromocytoma
  - Cushing's syndrome
  - Renin-secreting tumors
- Drugs
  - Cocaine, sympathomimetic agents, erythropoietin, cyclosporine

➤ **Treatment:**

The calcium channel blocker nicardipine is one of the few therapies used in the setting of hypertensive urgency. The usual oral dose is 30 mg, which can be repeated every 8 hours until the target blood pressure is achieved. Peak effect occurs within 10-20 minutes of dosing.

Labetalol has mixed α1- and β-adrenergic blocking properties and has an onset of action within 1 to 2 hours. The starting dose is 200 mg orally, which can be repeated every 3 to 4 hours to the desired blood pressure control.

Clonidine is a central sympatholytic (α2-adrenergic receptor agonist) agent with an onset of action within 15 to 30 minutes and a peak effect within 2 to 4 hours. A typical oral regimen is a 0.1 to 0.2 mg loading dose followed by 0.05 to 0.1 mg every hour until target blood pressure is achieved, up to a maximum dose of 0.7 mg. It can also be used as a transdermal agent or Catapres patch. Sudden discontinuation of clonidine may result in "rebound hypertension."

Hypertensive Emergency "Hypertensive Crises"

➢ **Definition:**

Hypertensive emergency (crisis) is characterized by a severe elevation in blood pressure complicated by impending or progressive target organ dysfunction. A hypertensive emergency is a situation in which uncontrolled hypertension is associated with acute end-organ damage. This could be a progression from the hypertensive urgency, or may develop *de novo*. There is often an associated acute coronary syndrome, stroke, and/ or renal failure.

➢ **Diagnosis:**

It requires a thorough history (evidence of target organ damage, illicit drug use, and medication compliance) as well as a complete physical examination, basic laboratory data, and electrocardiogram to assess for the presence of target organ damage and severity. Cocaine is often a culprit in the younger population, and a drug toxicology screen is recommended in the appropriate clinical setting.

➢ **Pathophysiology:**

Any disorder that causes hypertension can give rise to a hypertensive emergency. The rate of change in blood pressure determines the likelihood that an acute hypertensive syndrome will develop. Pre-existing chronic hypertension may lower the probability of a hypertensive emergency (at a particular blood pressure) through adaptive vascular changes that protect end organs from acute changes in blood pressure.

➤ **Causes (Similar to the Hypertensive Urgency):**
- Systemic or essential hypertension
- Renovascular disease
  - Acute glomerulonephritis
  - Vasculitis
  - Hemolytic uremic syndrome (HUS)
  - Thrombotic thrombocytopenic purpura (TTP)
  - Renal artery stenosis (RAS)
- Pregnancy
  - Eclampsia
- Endocrine
  - Pheochromocytoma
  - Cushing's syndrome
  - Renin-secreting tumors
- Drugs
  - Cocaine, sympathomimetic agents, erythropoietin, cyclosporine

➤ **Treatment (IV agents used in Hypertensive Emergencies):**
- **Nitroprusside**
  - Initial 0.3 (mg/kg)/min; usual 2–4 (mg/kg)/min; maximum 10 (mg/kg)/min for 10 min
- **Nicardipine**
  - Initial 5 mg/h; titrate by 2.5 mg/h at 5–15 min; max 15 mg/h
- **Enalaprilat**
  - Usual 0.625–1.25 mg over 5 min every 6–8 h; maximum 5 mg/dose
- **Esmolol**
  - Initial 80–500 mg/kg over 1 min, then 50–300 (mg/kg)/min

- **Phentolamine**
  - 5–15 mg bolus
- **Nitroglycerin**
  - Initial 5 mg/min, then titrate by 5 mg/min at 3–5 min intervals; if no response is seen at 20 mg/min, incremental increases of 10–20 mg/min may be used
- **Hydralazine**
  - 10–50 mg at 30-min intervals, to achieve the desired BP
- **Labetalol**
  2 mg/min up to 300 mg or 20 mg over 2 min, then 40–80 mg at 10-min intervals up to 300 mg total

* Constant blood pressure monitoring is required; hence an arterial line is indicated for the hemodynamic monitoring. Start with the lowest possible dose and titrate to achieve an optimal response. Subsequent dosing and intervals of administration should be adjusted according to the blood pressure response and duration of action of the specific agent.

Malignant Hypertension

➤ **Definition:**
This is defined as an abrupt increase in blood pressure in patients with chronic hypertension or sudden onset of severe hypertension. This is considered a medical emergency.

➤ **Pathophysiology:**
The most important factor leading to the development of malignant hypertension is a severe, rapid elevation of blood pressure. Because there is considerable overlap in the BP of patients with stable and malignant hypertension, other factors seem to be necessary to initiate the malignant phase.

➤ **Causes:**
- Essential hypertension
- Renal parenchymal etiologies

- Systemic disorders with renal involvement
  - Renovascular diseases
  - Systemic sclerosis
  - HUS/TFP
  - Diabetes mellitus
  - SLE
- Pheochromocytoma
- Conn's syndrome
- Cushing's syndrome
- Drugs
  - Cocaine
  - Amphetamines
  - Clonidine withdrawal
  - MAOI interactions
  - Erythropoietin
  - Cyclosporine
- Tumor-related
  - Renal cell carcinoma (RCC)
  - Wilms' tumor
  - Lymphoma
- Coarctation of the aorta

➢ **Symptoms:**
- Some of the common symptoms include:
  - Blurry vision
  - Chest pain
  - Seizure
  - Decreased urine output
  - Weakness or strange tingling/numbness in the arms, legs, or face
  - Headache
  - Shortness of breath

➢ **Treatment:**
- Nitroprusside
- Labetalol

- Nitroglycerin
- Trimethaphan
- Hydralazine
- Propranolol
- Phentolamine
- Captopril
- Nifedipine
- Minoxidil

Environmental Medicine and Temperature Regulation

1. Therapeutic Hypothermia/ Hypothermia Protocol (TH)
2. Hyperthermia
3. Malignant Hyperthermia
4. Heat Exhaustion
5. Heat Stroke
6. Frostnip and Frostbite
7. Near Drowning

Therapeutic Hypothermia (TH)

➤ **Definition:** Lowering the body temperature to 32-34 degree Celsius (89-93 F). TH is achieved to lower the metabolic demands of the central nervous system, by quickly lowering the body temperature. It can result in improved neurological outcomes in patients with cardiac arrest.
➤ **Indications:**
  ▪ Ventricular fibrillation (V-FIB)
  ▪ Ventricular tachycardia (V-TACH) witnessed cardiac arrest, with return of spontaneous circulation (ROSC) after the resuscitation efforts
➤ **Timing:** The clinical/neurological outcomes are much better if the hypothermia protocol is initiated soon after the cardiovascular insult. Ideally should be initiated within 6-8 hours

post cardiac arrest. Any absolute contraindications should be excluded prior to the protocol initiation.

➤ **Duration:** Time duration is calculated once target body temperature of 32 C is reached. The hypothermia (32 degrees Celsius) is maintained for 24 hours.

➤ **Relative Contraindications:**
- Major head trauma
- Major surgery within the past two weeks
- Septic shock, rule out infection by performing a CXR, obtaining cultures
- Coma due to metabolic causes, DKA, HONK, myxedema, or drugs (prescription or abuse)
- Bleeding disorders
- Brain death is suspected (CT head/MRI may be needed to rule out CVA)
- Certain lab values may also help prognosticate application of the TH protocol. Lactate level >11 in one study was associated with a poor survival rate.

➤ **Methods:**
- External cooling with blankets and ice. This is a conventional cooling strategy, first used by Hippocrates on wounded soldiers.
- Internal cooling with the Arctic Sun or Zoll Intravascular Temperature Management System (ITMS)
- A 9-10 French central venous catheter is placed in the femoral vein. It is longer than the usual central line and has coils surrounding its distal end, which help achieve the target temperature very efficiently.

➤ **Monitoring:**
- Arterial line for blood pressure monitoring and frequent blood draws for the ABGs
- Bladder and/or rectal temperature probe, with q1-2 monitoring

- Swan-Ganz catheter for hemodynamic/temperature monitoring
- Arrhythmia monitoring by continuous telemetry
- Central venous pressure (CVP) monitoring (keep MAP >70)
- Frequent blood work to assess and correct electrolyte status
- Skin checks q2 hours to look for skin burns, especially when using external cooling blankets
- "Train of Four" for the neurological monitoring with the goal to keep the patient 1-2 out of 4 (with 4 being the most sedated)

➢ **Medications:**
- Sedative (Precedex, propofol, Versed) and a neuromuscular blocking agent (Nimbex, succinylcholine) may be needed to control excessive shivering. These agents also provide ventilator synchrony especially when using the external cooling process. It becomes less important with the internal cooling method, since the target temperature is achieved rather quickly without significant shivering.

➢ **Rewarming:**
- Achieved as a passive process
- Initiated at 24 hours of the initiation of the protocol
- Maintain sedation/paralytics during this phase until the patient's body temperature reaches 36 C (97F)
- Watch for hypotension, as previously constricted capillaries can dilate and blood may pool in the lower extremities, resulting in decreased venous return
- Goal of rewarming is to achieve normothermia and avoid overshooting the target temperature, inducing hyperthermia, which is more deleterious
- Stop potassium infusions 8 hours prior to the rewarming phase

Hyperthermia

- ➢ **Definition:** Higher than normal body temperature. The normal temperature ranges up to 37 degree Celsius (98.6 F).
- ➢ **Classification:**
    - ▪ **Pathologic:** Febrile response to the infectious illness SIRS, sepsis, and systemic conditions such as connective tissue diseases, i.e., rheumatoid arthritis
    - ▪ **Environmental Exposures:** Heat exhaustion, heat stroke
    - ▪ **Therapeutic Hypothermia:** Induced hypothermia protocol in cardiac arrest patients. There can be inadvertent "overshoot hyperthermia" during the rewarming phase.
    - ▪ **Local Hyperthermia** (thermal ablation)
    - ▪ **Regional Hyperthermia** (Whole-body hyperthermia)
    - ▪ **Malignant Hyperthermia**
- ➢ **Heat Sources:**
    - ▪ Microwave
    - ▪ Radio-frequency wave (radio-frequency ablation or RFA) is the   most commonly used ablation method
    - ▪ Ultrasound wave
- ➢ **Application methods:**
    - ▪ External
    - ▪ Internal
- ➢ **Side Effects:**
    - ▪ **Local:** skin burns, soft tissue, nerve and muscle injury
    - ▪ **Systemic:** nausea, vomiting, diarrhea, dehydration, and organ dysfunction may occur
- ➢ **Clinical Uses:**
    - ▪ Cancer treatment for the solid organ tumors, lungs, breast, etc.

Malignant Hyperthermia

- ➢ **Definition:**

    It is an inherited condition characterized by a sudden rise in body temperature upon exposure to certain general anesthetic agents. It is associated with high-grade fever and muscle contractions.

➤ **Signs and Symptoms:**
- Body temperature >105 F
- Muscle stiffness and contractions
- Kidney failure due to accumulation of the muscle waste products myoglobin (rhabdomyolysis), i.e., pigment-induced nephropathy

➤ **Diagnosis:**
- Recent administration of the general anesthetic
- Determination of the renal functions and electrolytes
- Urine myoglobin
- Muscle biopsy

➤ **Treatment:**
- Supportive care, hydration, respiratory and hemodynamic support
- Prevention is the key
- Genetic counseling may be needed in susceptible families

Heat Exhaustion

➤ **Definition:** A clinical syndrome characterized by symptoms of dehydration and volume loss. It is caused by prolonged exposure to higher than normal external body temperatures. Excessive sweating or insensible heat loss is the key element behind the dehydration. The body temperature usually doesn't exceed 104 degrees Fahrenheit.

➤ **Symptoms:**
- Muscle cramps (charley horse) that occur due to electrolyte imbalance
- Pale but moist skin
- Excessive sweating
- Headache
- Excessive thirst
- Nausea and vomiting

➢ **Treatment:**
- Prevent exposure to heat
- Stop the physical activity
- Hydrate (orally or IV, if patient is obtunded, unconscious, or vomiting)
- Remove clothing, which allows for the heat dissipation
- Application of ice or water/immersion in cold water in severe cases

Heat Stroke (Sun Stroke)

➢ **Definition:** A life-threatening clinical condition caused by a sudden and often prolonged heat exposure. The body temperature often exceeds 105 degrees Fahrenheit. The increase in body temperature results in altered thermostatic regulation of the brain. There is loss of normal temperature control resulting in unregulated body temperature. It can be fatal if not immediately recognized and treated.

➢ **Symptoms:**
- Dehydration results in multiple organ dysfunction
  □ Central nervous system: confusion, seizures
  □ Cardiovascular: chest pain, tachycardia, low blood pressure, and syncope. Symptoms may mimic heart attack
  □ Respiratory: breathing difficulties, hyperventilation
  □ GI: abdominal pain, nausea, vomiting
  □ Skin: red, hot skin, often no associated sweating
  □ Renal: low urine output, electrolyte abnormalities, and renal failure may occur

➢ **Treatment:** *Cool the patient as soon as possible*
- Remove from the hot environment
- Rest
- Application of cool mist by a fan
- Immersion in cold water
- Don't give fluid to drink if mental status is altered or

patient has nausea/vomiting

- Achieve internal cooling by chilled intravenous fluid, bladder irrigation
- Monitor and correct electrolyte imbalances
- Monitor urine output
- In-patient treatment is often required
- Avoid alcohol or caffeinated beverages

Frostnip & Frostbite

➢ **Definition:** Tissue damage caused by exposure to an extreme cold environment. Frostnip is the milder version, whereas frostbite is a severe form of cold injury. If it is severe, it can result in tissue and organ damage/failure.

➢ **Symptoms:**
- Pain
- Paresthesia
- Blood clots (thrombosis of the extremities)
- Edema of the affected tissues
- Necrosis

➢ **Factors associated with worst outcomes:**
- Smoking
- Alcohol use
- Duration and degree of exposure
- Underlying co-morbid conditions such as PVD/CAD, Raynaud's disease

➢ **Diagnosis:**
- History and clinical exam
- X-ray
- Angiography
- Thermography

➢ **Treatment:**
- Environmental control (remove from the site of exposure)
- Remove wet, tight clothing

- Apply padding/splints when necessary
- Don't rub the affected area with snow
- Apply heat if rescue will be prolonged (>2 hours)
- Avoid freeze-thaw cycle
- Warm the affected area with warm water (>40 degrees Celsius) for 15 minutes
- Pain control
- If foreign bodies are found in the affected area, local debridement may be necessary
- Antibiotics, if suspect infection
- Tetanus vaccination/booster if patient has not been vaccinated in the past 10 years
- Hydrotherapy, physical and occupational therapy as needed in severe cases

➢ **Prevention:**
- Cover exposed surfaces (head, hands, and feet)
- Multiple layers of loose clothing
- Avoid smoking and alcohol, which can exacerbate the cold-related injury

Near Drowning

➢ **Definition:** It is a drowning event in which patient survives after being submerged underwater.

➢ **Symptoms:**
Respiratory symptoms: cough, shortness of breath, aspiration
Cardiac-related events: cardiac arrest, arrhythmias

➢ **Who is at risk:**
- Children may have near drowning in only a few inches of water
- Alcoholics
- Extreme winter/ice-related sports (ice fishing, skiing)
- Suicidal
- Accidental

➤ **Treatment:**
- Do not put yourself in danger, call for help
- Perform CPR when patient has cardiopulmonary arrest
- Stabilize neck
- Hospitalize if necessary
- Electrolyte monitoring and replacement

Neurologic Issues in Critical Care

1. Wernicke's Encephalopathy
2. Korsakoff's Syndrome
3. Nonconvulsive Status Epilepticus (NCSE)
4. Guillain-Barré Syndrome (GBS)
5. Miller-Fischer Syndrome (MFS)
6. Glasgow Coma Scale (GCS)
7. Brain Death
8. Apnea Test
9. PRESS Syndrome (Posterior Reversible Encephalopathy)
10. Syndrome of Inappropriate ADH Secretion (SIADH)
11. Diabetes Inspidus (DI)
12. Central DI
13. Nephrogenic DI
14. Cerebral Salt Wasting Syndrome (CSWS)
15. Intracranial Pressure Monitoring (ICP)
16. Brain Herniation Syndrome

Wernicke's Encephalopathy
 ➢ **Definition:**
  Reversible neurological state that results from thiamine (B1) deficiency
 ➢ **Etiology:**
  ▪ Alcoholism

- Hyperemesis gravidarum (excessive vomiting during pregnancy)
- ➢ **Differential Diagnosis:**
  - Phencyclidine (PCP) ingestion (no sedation, normal reflexes)
- ➢ **Clinical Diagnosis:**
  - Oculogyric crises
  - Altered consciousness (range from inebriation to obtundation)
  - Ataxia (unsteady gait)
  - Hyperreflexia
- ➢ **Labs (everything slows down):**
  - Hypoglycemia
  - Metabolic alkalosis
  - Hypokalemia
  - Hemoconcentration
  - Azotemia
  - Increased LFTs
- ➢ **Treatment:**
  - Thiamine should be administered before glucose or IV fluid infusion

Korsakoff's Syndrome

It is an irreversible neurological condition characterized by amnesia, confabulations, and lack of insight. This phenomenon can result when a reversible condition such as Wernicke's is not optimally treated. Most common reason is when glucose or IV fluid is infused prior to the thiamine administration in the susceptible population.

Nonconvulsive Status Epilepticus (NCSE)

- ➢ Encephalographic (EEG) evidence of seizure activity without obvious seizures (tonic-clonic). Prolonged NCSE (>30-60 min) can result in permanent neurologic injury.
- ➢ **Etiologies:**
  - Acute or traumatic brain injury (TBI)

- Following status epilepticus (8%)
- Infections/sepsis
- Half of the patients have preexisting seizure disorder/epilepsy
- 50% may have generalized tonic-clonic seizure at some point
- There may be an unexplained cause in some cases
- Cerebral tumors

➤ **Diagnosis:**
  - Continuous EEG/video monitoring
  - Brain CT/MRI scan

➤ **Treatment:**
  - Antiseizure (phenytoin-Keppra)/benzodiazepines/propofol and other antiseizure medications should be given with any clinical suspicion or evidence of seizure activity. Artificial coma with sedative and neuromuscular agents may be needed to achieve "seizure free status" in refractory cases.

Guillain-Barré Syndrome (GBS)

➤ **Definition:** Most common cause of acute generalized ascending paralysis
➤ **Classification:**
  - Acute inflammatory demyelinating polyneuropathy (AIDP)
  - Acute pan-pseudo autonomic type
  - Acute motor neuropathy
  - Overlap syndrome
➤ **Pathogenesis:**
  - Aberrant T-cell response to a prior infection that results in macrophage-induced destruction of the myelin sheath. Myelin sheath coats and protects the neuron from any external damage.
➤ **Pre-disposition:**
  - Flu like symptoms
  - Gastroenteritis with campylobacter jejuni

➤ **Signs/symptoms:**
  ▪ Symmetric ascending paralysis
  ▪ Paresthesia
  ▪ Hyperreflexia/arreflexia
  ▪ Respiratory failure due to diaphragmatic paralysis
➤ **Diagnosis:**
  ▪ Electromyography (EMG) shows axonal neuropathic/myopathic pattern
  ▪ Cerebrospinal fluid (CSF) shows no cells, increased protein content, and antiganglioside antibodies
  ▪ Muscle biopsy shows denervation atrophy
➤ **Treatment:**
  ▪ Plasmapheresis
  ▪ Intravenous immunoglobulin (IVIG)
  ▪ Supportive care, i.e., ventilatory or hemodynamic support
➤ **Differential Diagnosis:**
  ▪ Critical illness polyneuropathy
    ▫ It is an acute sensorimotor deficit that affects lower extremity in critically ill patients.
    ▫ Caused by microcirculatory damage due to decreased perfusion or endothelial injury from cytokine mediated inflammatory response. Axonal degeneration is noted on EMG.
  ▪ Critical illness myopathy
    ▫ Acute muscular weakness, resulting in paralysis in critically ill patients
    ▫ May occur with critical illness polyneuropathy
    ▫ Caused by sepsis, multi-organ failure
    ▫ Presents as *"failure to wean"* in mechanically ventilated patients
    ▫ Flaccid paralysis
    ▫ Usually spares the cranial nerves

Miller-Fischer Syndrome (MFS)

> ➢ Less common variant of the GBS
> ➢ Triad
>   ▪ Opthalmoplegia
>   ▪ Ataxia
>   ▪ Decreased or absent reflexes
> ➢ Typical ascending paralysis is absent
> ➢ Acute phase is mediated by IgG antibodies
> ➢ Cranial nerves are involved, contrary to GBS
> ➢ Predisposing factors
>   ▪ Viral GI illness
>   ▪ Bacterial GI illness, esp. campylobacter spp.
>   ▪ HIV/AIDS
>   ▪ Hodgkin's disease
>   ▪ Recent immunizations
> ➢ Treatment
>   ▪ Immunoglobulin-G (IgG)
>   ▪ Plasmapheresis

Glasgow Coma Scale (GCS)

Mnemonic: EVM

> ➢ **Best score - 15**
>   ▪ E (eyes)   4   spontaneous eye opening
>   ▪ V (verbal)   5   verbally oriented
>   ▪ M (Motor)   6   obeys command
> ➢ **Severity**
>   ▪ 13 - 15 is mild injury
>   ▪ 9 - 12 is moderate injury
>   ▪ <8 is severe injury
> ➢ **GCS <8**
>   ▪ Often associated with an increased intracranial pressure (ICP)
>   ▪ ICP monitoring may be indicated in selective group of patients

- GCS is a less reliable prognostic tool in patients with non-traumatic brain injury
- Limited value in sedated patients
- Best GCS score for the intubated patient is 10 (T). "T" stands for intubated, since verbal orientation can't be assessed due to the endotracheal tube.

Brain Death

➢ **Definition:** Permanent absence of cerebral and brainstem functions
➢ **Prerequisites:**
  - Appropriate clinical setting
    □ Trauma
    □ Structural pathology on brain imaging
      − Subarachnoid hemorrhage (SAH)
      − Intracranial hemorrhage (ICH)
      − Cerebrovascular accidents (CVA-stroke)
    □ Hypoxic/ischemic encephalopathy
      − Prolonged cardiopulmonary arrest
    □ Neurologic exam
      − Absent cerebral brainstem function
      − Apnea test positive
➢ **Confounding Variables (must exclude):**
  - Acid-base disturbance or extreme electrolyte imbalances
  - Endocrine disorder, myxedema coma, hypothyroidism
  - Drug overdose or poisoning
  - Central nervous system (CNS) disorders
  - Neuromuscular (NM) blockade
  - Deep sedation
  - Hypothermia (<37 C)

Apnea Test

➢ **Definition:**

Test performed on the intubated and mechanically ventilated patient to assess spontaneous breathing ability

  ➢ **Performed to Assess Brain Death:**
- Pre-oxygenate with 100% O2 for 10 minutes
- Check ABGs at baseline
- Disconnect from the ventilator
- Continuous O2 is provided by tracheal catheter with the tip approximated near the carina, for 6-8 minutes
- Patient observed for 8-10 minutes

  ➢ **Positive Test:**
- No observed spontaneous breaths associated with a rise in the PaCO2 greater than 60 or >20 mmHg increase over the baseline carbon dioxide level determined by ABGs

  ➢ **Situations in Which Apnea Test Can Be Done:**
- Hypothermia
- Vasopressor use

  ➢ **Complications:**
- Desaturation, leading up to further neurological injury
- Arrhythmia, V-Tachycardia, V-Fib, SVT
- These complications should be addressed with the family prior to the apnea test, as these may have long-term implications

  ➢ **Alternatives to the Apnea Test:**
- Electroencephalogram (EEG), usually is non-specific
- Brain-evoked potentials
- Cerebral angiography
- Brain scan/ Doppler scan (nuclear medicine)

PRESS Syndrome (Posterior Reversible Encephalopathy)

  ➢ **Definition:** Characterized by acute mental status changes, mimicking stroke, which is associated with uncontrolled hypertension

➤ **Clinical Features:**
  ▪ Change in mental status
  ▪ Uncontrolled blood pressure
  ▪ Stroke-like symptoms
➤ **Pathogenesis:**
  ▪ Caused by uncontrolled hypertension, eclampsia, and drugs, i.e., tacrolimus
➤ **Diagnosis:**
  ▪ Magnetic Resonance Imaging (MRI)
➤ **Treatment:**
  ▪ Blood pressure control
  ▪ Withdrawal of medication, if that is the underlying pathology
➤ **Prognosis:**
  Usually reversible with the correction of the underlying cause, such as optimal blood pressure control or discontinuing the culprit medication

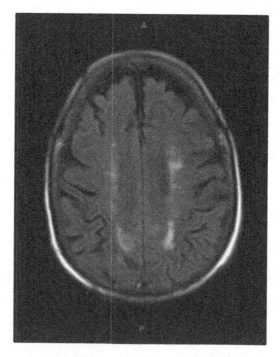

Syndrome of Inappropriate ADH Secretion (SIADH)

➢ **Definition:**

Levels of ADH are inappropriately elevated compared to body's low osmolality, and the ADH levels are not suppressed by further decreases in osmolality.

➢ **Etiology:**

- **Irritation of CNS:** meningitis, encephalitis, brain tumors, brain hemorrhage, hypoxic insult, trauma, brain abscess, Guillain-Barré syndrome, hydrocephalus
- **Pulmonary disorders:** pneumonia, asthma, positive pressure ventilation (PPV), cystic fibrosis (CF), tuberculosis (TB), pneumothorax
- **Drugs:** vincristine, vinblastine, opiates, carbamazepine, cyclophosphamide
- **Paraneoplastic syndrome:** These produce ectopic ADH-like peptides: oat cell lung carcinoma, Ewing's sarcoma, carcinoma of duodenum, pancreas, and thymus

➢ **Functions of ADH:**

- Antidiuretic hormone (ADH) = vasopressin=opposite of diuresis. It helps retain water
- ADH is synthesized in the supra-optic nuclei in the hypothalamus and stored in the posterior pituitary
- Normally released into the bloodstream when osmo-receptors detect high plasma osmolality
- At the kidney level, ADH binds to its receptors in the collecting ducts, opening water channels
- Water is passively reabsorbed along the kidney's medullary concentration gradient

➢ **Signs and Symptoms:**

- Decreases urine output and retains water
- Signs of hyponatremia (same amount of sodium dissolved in more water): lethargy, apathy, disorientation, muscle cramps, anorexia, and agitation
- Signs of water toxicity: nausea, vomiting, personality

changes, confusion, and combativeness

- If Na < 110 mEq/L, seizures, bulbar palsies, hypothermia, stupor, coma may ensue

➤ **Laboratory Values:**

- Serum Na < 135 because sodium is diluted by excessive free water reabsorption
- Serum osmolality low (normal is ~ 270)
- Urine Na is inappropriately high, >20 mmol/L, actually losing Na in urine instead of retaining it
- Urine osmolality is inappropriately high, can range between 300-1400 mosm/L
- CVP is high due to free water retention

➤ **Treatment:**

- Fluid restriction, ¾ of maintenance fluids
- If symptomatic, may actually need to replace sodium chloride. Hypertonic saline can be used, for example: 300 cc/m2 of 1½ % NS
- Diuretics such as Lasix or Bumex
- Treat the underlying disorder and the SIADH will usually resolve (for example, after surgical removal of lung carcinomas)
- Demeclochlorotetracycline (tetracycline antibiotic) blocks ADH receptors in the renal collecting ducts
- Hemodialysis in severe cases
- WARNING: if sodium is corrected too fast, there is a risk of central pontine myelinolysis (CPM) or brain herniation
- Maximum correction of sodium should be limited to 15 mEq over 24 hours

Diabetes Insipidus (DI)

➤ **Definition:** It is a clinical condition characterized by inability to effectively conserve urinary water

➤ **Types:**

- **Central:** ADH not synthesized or not released from the

hypothalamic- pituitary axis

- **Nephrogenic:** ADH is released normally but not detected by the receptors in the collecting ducts of the kidney. It can also present as a sex-linked recessive condition. Other causes include renal disease, electrolyte disorders, and some medication side effects.

➤ **Etiology:**
- Head trauma
- Brain neoplasms
- Congenital CNS defects
- CNS infections
- CNS hypoxia
- ADH secretion is decreased by certain drugs: alcohol, Demerol, morphine, Dilantin, barbiturates, glucocorticoids

➤ **Signs and Symptoms:**
- Polyuria
- Polydipsia
- Electrolyte imbalance

Central Diabetes Insipidus (Central DI)

➤ **Definition:**

Central DI is caused by a decreased or absent secretion of the ADH from the posterior pituitary. This results in polyuria, dehydration, and electrolyte abnormalities.

- Dehydration may not be readily apparent because of hyperosmolality and fluid shifts. The fluid moves from the extracellular compartment to intravascular spaces, therefore maintaining optimal blood pressure control.
- Weight loss is a better measure of fluid status than determination of the hemodynamic status

➤ **Lab Values:**
- Hypernatremia, Na > 150-160
- High serum osmolality (normal 270)
- Urine Na < 20 mmol/L

- Low urine osmolality (very dilute urine)
➤ **Treatment:**
  - Increase oral or intravenous free water consumption
  - May use hypotonic saline to dilute the relative hypernatremia
  - Volume replacement volume for volume (<u>cc</u> for <u>cc</u>)
  - Vasopressin/ADH administration (bolus or drip 1.5-2.5 mU/kg/hr)
  - Treating the underlying cause

Cerebral Salt Wasting Syndrome (CSWS)

➤ **Definition:** Extreme hyponatremia and dehydration associated with brain injury, hemorrhage, or a tumor. This condition results from the loss of sodium from the renal tubules, hence the term "salt wasting caused by centrally mediated causes."

Etiology:
  - Closed head injury
  - CNS surgery
  - CNS tumors
  - CNS infections, meningitis

➤ **Signs and Symptoms:**
  - Polyuria (>2 liters in the first 24 hours), with polydipsia
  - Weight loss
  - Dehydration/hypovolemic
  - Orthostatic hypotension
  - Low CVP because of low circulating blood volume
  - Craving for high-salt food

➤ **Laboratory Values:**
  - Hyponatremia due to excessive renal sodium loss
  - High urine Na > 20 mmol/L
  - Increased plasma atrial natriuretic peptide (ANP) because of low circulating volume
  - Inappropriately normal or low aldosterone and ADH levels despite high ANP levels

➢ **Treatment:**
- Volume for volume replacement of the urine sodium losses
- When discharged from the hospital, most patients will need oral sodium supplementation
- Supplementation of fludrocortisone (Florinef), which is a mineralocorticoid, may be required in some patients

Intracranial Pressure (ICP) Monitoring

➢ **Physiology:**
- Normal: ICP < 15 mmHg in adults
- Intracranial hypertension: ICP> 20 mmHg
- Lower ICP in children than adults
- Sub atmospheric in newborns
- Protected by a rigid "Skull"
- Internal volume of 1400-1700 cc
- Intracranial contents (volume):
  - Brain parenchyma (80%)
  - CSF (10 %)
  - Blood (10 %)

➢ **Elevated ICP:**

Physiologic causes:
- Sneezing
- Coughing
- Valsalva maneuvers

Pathologic causes:
- Intracranial hemorrhage (ICH) and traumatic brain injury (TBI)
- Central nervous system infections
- Neoplasm
- Vasculitis
- Ischemic infarcts
- Hydrocephalus
- Pseudotumor cerebri

> **Flow of the Cerebrospinal Fluid:**
>   - Produced at a rate of approximately 20 mL/h (500 mL/day).
>   - Ependymal cells of the choroid plexus in the lateral ventricles produce CSF. It flows to the third ventricle and fourth ventricle via the foramen of Monro and aqueduct of Sylvius. Then it flows to the subarachnoid space and spinal cord through the foramen of Magendie and Luschka, and then to the fourth ventricle.
>   - Problems with CSF regulation generally result from:
>   □ Impaired outflow due to ventricular obstruction
>   □ Venous congestion may occur with venous sinus thrombosis, i.e., sagittal thrombosis
> **Intracranial Compliance:**
>   - There is interrelationship between changes in the volume of intracranial contents and ICP
>   - Intracranial compliance is equal to the change in volume over the change in pressure
>   Compliance = dV/dP

Kelly-Monroe Paradigm

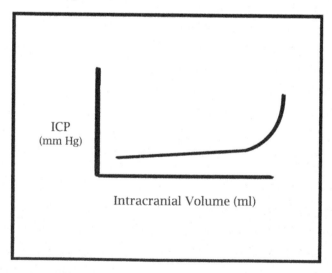

An initial increase in volume results in a small increase in pressure because of intracranial compensation (initial straight line). Further increases in intracranial volume result in a rise in ICP (curved line).

➢ **Clinical Manifestation:**
- Headache due to the pain fibers of CN-V
- Change in level of consciousness
- Vomiting
- CN VI palsy
- Periorbital bruising
- Cushing's Triad, also referred to as Cushing's Reflex (suggest increased ICP)
  - Hypertension
  - Bradycardia
  - Irregular respiration

Brain Herniation Syndrome

➢ **Definition:**
A potentially fatal disease caused by an increase in the ICP. It is usually associated with stroke, cerebral hemorrhage, trauma, contusion, or cerebral tumors.

➢ **Classification of herniation syndromes (anatomic):**
- Subfalcial (cingulate)
- Uncal
- Downward (central)
- External
- Tonsillar

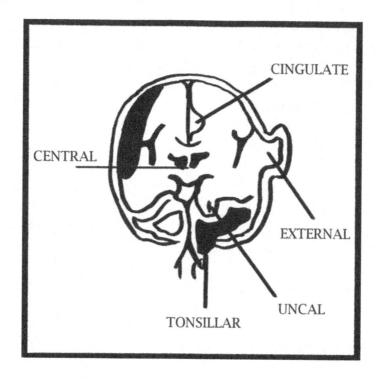

> **Sign/symptoms:**
> - Dilation of ipsilateral pupil
> - Hemiparesis
> - Cranial nerve III palsy
>   - **i.** Ptosis
>   - **ii.** Loss of medial gaze
> **Indications for ICP Monitoring:**
> - Closed head injury
> - Stroke (CVA)
> - Intracerebral hemorrhage (ICH)
> - Hydrocephalus
> - Subarachnoid hemorrhage (SAH)
> - Hepatic encephalopathy
> - Sagittal sinus thrombosis
> - Comatose head injury patients with GCS 3 to 8

- Abnormal cranial findings on CT
- Comatose patients with normal CT if they have:
  - Age >40 years
  - Unilateral or bilateral motor posturing
  - Systolic blood pressure <90 mmHg

Intracranial Pressure Monitors

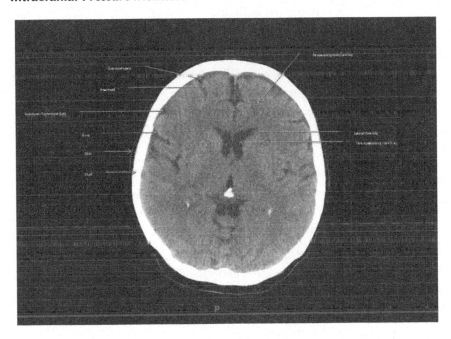

- ➤ Placement of the ICP monitors:
  - Intraparenchymal
  - Intraventricular
  - Subdural
  - Epidural
- ➤ Goals of ICP monitoring:
  - Keep ICP < 20 mmHg
  - Keep cerebral perfusion pressure CPP between 60 and 75 mmHg:
  - Maintains cerebral perfusion

- Prevents ischemic brain injury
- Improves clinical outcome
- Intervene when ICP > 20 mmHg for >5 to 10 minutes
- Brief elevation in ICP may occur due to the following:
  - Coughing
  - Movement
  - Suctioning
  - Ventilator asynchrony

➢ **General Management:**
- Treat the underlying cause
- Head elevation >30-40 degrees
- Intravenous mannitol
- Intubation if necessary
- Avoid depolarizing neuromuscular blocking agents (NMB), i.e., succinylcholine
- Use lidocaine, 4% for coughing
- Hyperventilation by increasing the minute ventilation (respiratory rate or tidal volume) on the ventilator. Keeping the PCO_2 in the 24-26 range causes vasoconstriction, thereby decreasing the ICP. This, however, is a temporary measure, since the vasoconstriction may last for a short period.

➢ **Fluid Management:**
- No fluid restriction
- Keep euvolemic and iso-osmolar to hyperosmolar
- Use isotonic saline 0.9 % saline
- Avoid all free water
  - D5W
  - 0.45 % saline
  - Enteral free water
- Serum osmolality should be kept >280 mOsm/L (295 - 305 mOsm/L)
- Colloid versus crystalloid
  - Colloids, i.e., albumin offers no additional benefit,

rather have been found to be detrimental compared with the NS/LR

- Hypertonic saline
  - Bolus doses may acutely lower ICP
  - No long-term benefits

➤ **Sedation:**
- Decrease ICP by:
- Reducing metabolic demand
- Preventing ventilator asynchrony
- Sympathetic responses of hypertension and tachycardia
- Precedex or propofol can be used for sedation:
  - Easily titratable & short half-life
  - Permits frequent neurologic assessment

➤ **Patient Positioning:**
- Reduce excessive flexion or rotation of the neck
- Minimize stimuli that can cause Valsalva response
- Head elevated above the heart (usually >30 degrees) to increase venous outflow, as long as the CPP remains between 70-90

➤ **Fever:**
- Elevates brain metabolism
- Increases cerebral blood flow (CBF)
- Elevates ICP by increasing the volume of blood in the cranial vault
- Aggressively treat fever with:
  - Acetaminophen
  - Cooling devices

➤ **Antiseizure Measures:**
- Seizures can worsen the ICP
- Treat promptly and aggressively, if seizures are suspected or witnessed
- High-risk mass lesions (supratentorial cortical locations)
- Lesions adjacent to the cortex (subdural hematoma or subarachnoid hemorrhage)

- **Mannitol** is an osmotic diuretic that reduces brain volume by drawing free water out of the tissue and into the circulation and forcing subsequent diuresis
- Doses
- Bolus of 1 g/kg IV
  - Repeat doses at 0.25 to 0.5 g/kg Q6H as needed

➤ **Corticosteroids:**

Not useful in the management of:
- Infarction
- Intracranial hemorrhage

Useful in the management of:
- Brain tumors
- CNS infections

➤ **Hyperventilation:**
- Lowers $PaCO_2$
- Keep $PaCO_2$ between 26-30 mmHg
- Rapidly reduces ICP through vasoconstriction
- 1 mmHg change in $PaCO_2$ is associated with 3 % change in CBF
- Should be careful in the acute stroke setting

➤ **Therapeutic Hypothermia:**
- Hypothermia decreases cerebral metabolism and reduces CBF and ICP
  - Maintain the core body temperature between 32 to 33°C following traumatic brain injury to decrease mortality and improve neurologic outcome

➤ **Decompressive Craniotomy "Burr Holes":**
- Removes the rigid confines of the bony skull
- Craniotomy alone lowers ICP by 15%
- Craniotomy plus opening the dura lowers ICP by 70%

Intracranial Hemorrhage

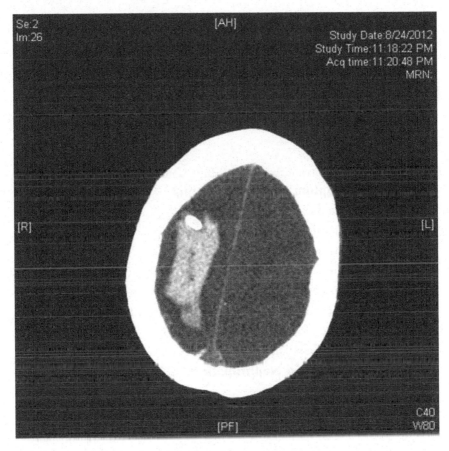

Renal/Electrolyte Abnormalities

1. Acute Symptomatic Hyponatremia
2. Calciphylaxis
3. Acid/Base Disturbances (ABGs)
4. Caveats of Bicarbonate Infusion
5. Acute Renal Failure/Acute Kidney Injury (AKI)
6. Indications for Hemodialysis
7. Chronic Renal Replacement Therapy (CCRT) or Continuous Veno-Venous Hemofiltration (CVVH)
8. Rhabdomyolysis
9. Contrast-Induced Nephropathy (CIN)

Acute Symptomatic Hyponatremia

➢ **Definition:**
  ▪ Low serum sodium level, which is associated with neurological and clinical sequalae
➢ **Symptoms:**
  ▪ Nausea, vomiting, headache, muscle weakness, cramps, confusion, lethargy, seizure (varies with the sodium levels and the chronicity of the disease)
➢ **Radiology:**
  ▪ +/- Acute cerebral edema (effacement of cortical sulci-CT/MRI)
➢ **Duration:**
  ▪ <24 hours is acute, >48 hours is chronic

- ➤ **Risk of Central Pontine Myelinolysis (CPM):**
  - ▪ Low with acute asymptomatic hyponatremia
  - ▪ More likely with acute symptomatic hyponatremia
- ➤ **Treatment:**
  - ▪ It is a medical emergency
  - ▪ Treatment is directed towards the underlying cause
  - ▪ Increase sodium by 2 mmol/hr (maximum 12mEq/day) until symptomatic resolution and sodium correction
  - ▪ Can use 3% or 5% of hypertonic saline in patients with symptomatic hyponatremia such as seizure
  - ▪ Once target sodium level is achieved, a free water restriction of 500-1000 mL/day should be continued until complete resolution

Calciphylaxis
- ➤ **Definition:**
  - ▪ Rare condition characterized by abnormal calcium deposition, resulting in the occlusion of small arterioles, tissue hypoperfusion, and organ ischemia
  - ▪ It is a form of dystrophic calcification
- ➤ **Risk Factors:**
  - ▪ End-stage renal disease (ESRD)
  - ▪ Obesity
  - ▪ Decreased albumin
  - ▪ Coumadin administration
  - ▪ Critical illness, sepsis, respiratory failure
- ➤ **Sequalae:**
  - ▪ Ischemic necrosis of fat and muscle
  - ▪ Painful subcutaneous nodules or calcified plaques
  - ▪ Ischemic ulcers
  - ▪ Sepsis syndrome, which may lead to death
- ➤ **Diagnosis:**
  - ▪ Biopsy shows arteriolar calcification and occlusion. The biopsy site may become a nidus for an infection

> **Differential Diagnosis:**
> - Skin necrosis associated with protein C deficiency
> **Treatment:**
> - Supportive
> - Treatment of the underlying cause

Acid Base Disturbances (ABGs)

> ABG results should be interpreted in a systemic fashion. Stop at each step, understand the problem, and move to the next step.
> - pH shows acidosis or alkalosis
> - Is it a metabolic or respiratory problem?
> - If respiratory, is it acute or chronic?
> - If metabolic, is there respiratory compensation?
> - If metabolic acidosis, check anion gap (AG). Is it AG vs. non-anion gap (NAG)?
> - If AG metabolic acidosis, check delta gap
> With that in mind, let's begin:
> - pH (7.4)
>
> Acidosis <7.4
>
> Alkalosis >7.4
> - pCO2 (40)
>
> Metabolic (pH and pCO2 same direction)
>
> Respiratory (opposite direction)
> - If respiratory is it acute or chronic?
> - If metabolic AG or non-AG?
> - Compensation
> **Metabolic Acidosis**
> - Increase acid accumulation
> - Decreased bicarbonate level
> - Types:
>
>   **Anion Gap (AG)**
>
>   **Non-Anion Gap (NAG)**
> - **1-Anion Gap Metabolic Acidosis**

Definition AG>12

Differential **MUDPILES** (methanol, uremia, DKA, paraldehyde, INH, lactic acidosis, ethanol, and salicylates)

Diagnosis renal, lactate, ketones, osmolar gap

ASA, ETOH, drug toxicology screen

Treatment underlying cause

- **Lactic Acidosis**
  - Type A
    Tissue hypoperfusion (sepsis, low circulating blood volume)
  - Type B
    Cellular/mitochondrial dysfunction (toxicity of medications)
- **Osmolar Gap**
  - Measured osmolality-calculated osmolality
    - Calculated osmolality= $2 \times Na + BUN/2.8 + gluc/18$ (or sodium times two)
    - >20 suggest ingestion of ETOH ingestion
    - Ethanol, methanol, ethylene glycol
    - Isopropyl ETOH (normal electrolytes, acetone-urine)
- **Drugs That May Cause Metabolic Acidosis**
  - Metformin (in renal insufficiency)
  - HIV medication
  - Linezolid (Zyvox)
  - Preservative used in lorazepam (Ativan) can cause propylene glycol toxicity with high dose and prolonged use
  - Propofol-related infusion syndrome (PRIS)
- **Significance of Albumin in Calculating the AG**
  - For every decrease in albumin by 1 gram, there is a decrease of AG by 3
    (Paraproteinemia, i.e., multiple myeloma [MM], Waldenstrom's macroglobulinemia [WM]).
    Normal albumin level is 4.

- ▫ In alkalosis (pH >7.5), albumin becomes more negatively charged, so you can have an increased AG in the absence of acidosis
  - **Respiratory Compensation**
    - ▫ Expected CO2 (Winter's formula)
      1.5 x HCO3 + 8 (+/- 2)
    - ▫ Now calculate AG
      Normal 12

➤ **Non-Anion Gap Metabolic Acidosis**
- Definition Loss of bicarbonate, accumulation of chloride
- Differential GI diarrhea
  Renal loss of HCO3
- Diagnosis Urine gap=(Na+K)-Cl
  Positive gap=RTA
  Negative gap=diarrhea
- **Renal Tubular Acidosis (RTA)**
  - ▫ Check serum K level
  - ▫ If K level is high, it is type RTA-4
  - ▫ If K level is low
    - – Check urine pH
      If urine pH >5.5 distal RTA   (Type 1)
      If urine pH <5.5 proximal RTA   (Type 2)

RTA TYPES

Type 1 Distal
        Urine pH >5.5
        Bicarbonate =1-2 meq/kg/d
Type 2 Proximal
        Urine pH <5.5
        Bicarbonate=10-15 meq/kg/d
Type 3 Aldosterone deficiency or resistance
        If K is elevated, measure aldosterone level
        No bicarbonate infusion if hyperkalemia is treated

➢ **Metabolic Alkalosis**
- **Diagnosis**
  Urine chloride
  >20: Hypervolemic or chloride resistant
  - ▫ **Hypertension**
    (Mineralocorticoids retain Na, lose H and K)
    Primary hyperaldosteronism
    Liddle's syndrome
    Black European licorice
    11-17-beta hydroxylase deficiency
  - ▫ **Normal BP**
    Barter's syndrome
    Re-feeding syndrome
- **Treatment:** Underlying cause

➢ **Respiratory Acidosis**
- **Signs/Symptoms**
  CNS   headache, blurry vision, restlessness, anxiety
  CO2   narcosis, tremors, astrexis, delirium, somnolence
- **Differential Diagnosis**
  Depressed respiratory center, located in the medulla
  a) **Drugs:** opiates, anesthetic, sedative
  b) **Central Sleep Apnea**
  Obstruction of upper airway (OSA, aspiration)
  Impaired respiratory muscles and chest wall, i.e., polio, ALS, GBS
  Impaired alveolar gas exchange
  (COPD, ARDS, pulmonary edema, pneumothorax)
- **Diagnosis**
  pH <7.4 and PCO2 >40
- **Calculate A-a gradient** (normal 10-20)
  PaO2 = 150-(pCO2/0.8)
  A-a gradient >20 suggests intrinsic pulmonary diseases
- **Compensation**
  Acute: for every 10-mmHg increase in PCO2

plasma HCO3 increases by 1 meq/lit
(HCO3 max 30-33)
Chronic: for every 10 mmHg increase in PCO2
plasma HCO3 increases by 3 meq/lit
(Maximum HCO3 concentration goes to 45, since the kidney has time compensate)

➢ **Respiratory Alkalosis**
  ▪ **Diagnosis**
    pH >7.4 and PCO2 <40
  ▪ **Compensation**
    Acute   for every 10 mmHg decrease in PCO2
         plasma HCO3 decreases by 2 meq/lit
    Chronic for every 10 mmHg decrease in PCO2
         plasma HCO3 decreases by 4 meq/lit
         (pH can return to normal)
      ▫ *Respiratory alkalosis has even numbers for compensation. The bicarbonate changes by 2 in an acute setting and by 4 in the chronic setting.*

➢ **Mixed Metabolic Disorders**
  ▪ Calculate delta gap
    Calculate gap-12
  ▪ Calculate corrected plasma HCO3
    Plasma HCO3+delta AG
  ▪ If corrected plasma HCO3 >26
    Concomitant metabolic alkalosis
  ▪ If corrected plasma HCO3 <26
    Concomitant non-AG metabolic acidosis

➢ **Mixed Respiratory and Metabolic Disorders**
  ▪ Calculate expected pCO2 (metabolic acidosis)
    Winter's formula 1.5x HCO3+8 +/-2
  ▪ Faster method
    HC03 +15
      ▫ if measured PCO2> expected PCO2 (respiratory acidosis)

> □ if measured PCO2< expected PCO2 (respiratory alkalosis)

➤ **Triple Acid Base Disorders**
>   □ Metabolic acidosis+metabolic alkalosis+Respiratory acidosis or alkalosis
> ■ Examples
>   □ Diabetic ketoacidosis (DKA)
>   □ Alcohol
>   □ Aspirin
>   **Base Deficit**
> ■ The amount of acid or a base added to one liter of solution to normalize the pH to 7.4
> ■ Ignores the PCO2 (constant at 40)
> ■ Least reliable method of acid base disturbance because pCO2 is not included in the calculation

➤ **Stewart's Equation**
Most accurate method of acid/base calculation
> ■ PCO2
> ■ Weak acid (phosphate+albumin)
> ■ Strong ion difference

Sum of all strong cations minus strong anions
(K+Ca+Mg)-(Cl+other anions) Normal Range is 38-42

decrease	acidosis
increase	alkalosis

Caveats of Bicarbonate Replacement
> ■ Fluid overload
> ■ Electrolyte abnormalities
> ■ Intracellular acidosis
> ■ No change in the final clinical outcome
> ■ Tissue hypoxia
> ■ Overshoot alkalemia
> ■ Not used in the ACLS protocol due to lack of efficacy

Acute Renal Failure or Acute Kidney Injury (AKI)

➤ **Definition:**

- A sudden decline in glomerular filtration by the kidneys. This is caused by a host of factors that can cause kidney injury. It is characterized by an abrupt rise in the markers of blood urea nitrogen (BUN) and creatinine. The glomerular filtration rate (GFR) drops quite precipitously due to the kidney injury.

➤ **Etiology:**

- Acute tubular necrosis (ATN)
- Medications, i.e., NSAIDs, metformin (nephrotoxic agents)
- Trauma
- Rhabdomyolysis
- Shock (septic, cardiogenic, hypovolemic)

➤ **Pathogenesis:**

Blood flow to the kidney is reduced as a consequence of the initial insult. Blood pressure may be within normal range during the initial injury period. However, diminished blood flow ultimately results in release of pro-inflammatory cytokines, which results in the renal tubular damage. Since the tubular cells become ischemic during this time, they slough off and cause further obstruction of the renal tubules. This phenomenon compromises the renal flow and results in the reduced GFR.

➤ **Categories/Classification:**

There are generally three broad categories under which AKI can be described. These are pre-renal, renal, and post-renal. However, it can also be classified into oliguric and non-oliguric based on the urine output. The most commonly used criteria to classify acute renal failure is the RIFLE system (Risk, Injury, Failure, Loss of kidney function, and End-Stage Renal Disease or ESRD).

- **Pre-renal:** Volume depletion due to cardiac causes or hypovolemia. The BUN/creatinine ratio is elevated from the baseline of 10:1 to 20:1. Other causes of pre-renal disease include sepsis, anaphylaxis, drugs, CHF, liver cirrhosis, hypotension.

- **Renal or Intrinsic:** Kidney diseases caused by structural or functional abnormalities. The BUN/creatinine ratio is 10:1(normal range). Some of the conditions are glomerular diseases, vascular disease, rhabdomyolysis, drugs, infections, and systemic illness.

- **Post-renal:** Mostly obstructive in nature and caused by BPH, stones, strictures, or tumors. The BUN/creatinine ratio is 10:2. Abdominal compartment syndrome is another result of the pigment-induced nephropathy and ATN.

- **Oliguric vs. Non-Oliguric status:** This classification is based on the urine output. Most patients with acute renal failure present with non-oliguric state (still able to maintain good urine output).

- **Acute or Chronic Renal Failure:** It is the worsening of the pre-existing renal function.

Indications for Hemodialysis

➢ Acute/chronic or end-stage renal failure (ESRD)
➢ Severe fluid overload, resulting in pulmonary edema, respiratory distress or failure
➢ Profound electrolyte imbalances, i.e., hyperkalemia
➢ Drug overdose (drugs that are dialyzable, i.e., lithium, vancomycin)
➢ Refractory hypertension
➢ Pericarditis (pericardial rub may be auscultated)
➢ Severe metabolic acidosis
➢ Bleeding diathesis due to uremia
➢ Profound vomiting caused by electrolyte imbalance and uremia

Continuous Veno-Venous Hemofiltration (CVVH) or Continuous Renal Replacement Therapy (CRRT)

It is a temporary form of hemodialysis offered to critically ill patients with renal failure, and often initiated in the ICU setting. These patients are hemodynamically unstable and will not be able to tolerate conventional hemodialysis. The conventional mode of hemodialysis requires optimal blood pressure to maintain the filtration through the semipermeable membrane. The CVVH is managed by a consulting nephrologist. The ICU nurse usually operates the CVVH machine.

There are variations of this treatment modality. It is usually done through the venous system after inserting a dialysis catheter into the femoral, jugular, or subclavian vein. It offers the choice of running through the arterial system and returning the blood to the venous system. This variety is called veno-arterial hemofiltration (CVAH). *SCUF* is another term, meaning the *slow, continuous ultrafiltration of fluid*. This is done in surgical patients who have normal renal function and acid base status, but require fluid removal only. Since most of these patients are hypotensive or hemodynamically unstable, the goal of fluid removal is achieved rather slowly by CVVH.

Rhabdomyolysis

➢ **Definition:**

It is caused by destruction of the skeletal muscles with resultant renal failure. Myoglobin is the structural protein released as a result of the muscle breakdown.

➢ **Pathophysiology:**

It is a type of pigment-induced nephropathy. Accumulation of these proteins in the renal tubules causes renal failure.

➢ **Etiology:**

- Strenuous, unaccustomed, or eccentric exercise in untrained athletes and military recruits after prolonged marching in an austere environment
- Medications, i.e., statins, anesthetics

- Alcohol, certain toxins, and recreational substances like cocaine
- Extreme exposure to temperatures, i.e., heat stroke
- Crush injuries/trauma/electrical shock/lightning strike/ burns
- Prolonged immobilization in alcoholics, or the elderly after a fall
- Infections, viral infections

➢ **Sign and symptoms:**
  - Muscle pain
  - Tea-colored urine
  - Oliguria to anuria

➢ **Diagnosis:**
  - Clinical context, and may range from a subclinical picture manifested by elevated myoglobin to acute renal failure
  - Elevated creatinine phosphokinase (CPK) by dipstick urine

➢ **Complications:**
  - Acute renal failure
  - Electrolyte imbalance
  - Arrhythmias or cardiac arrest
  - Compartment syndrome, if there is only extremity involvement
  - DIC

➢ **Treatment:**
  - Aggressive intravenous volume resuscitation 1-2 liters/hr. Bicarbonate infusion is often used when associated with metabolic acidosis.
  - Maintain urine output >300cc/hr.
  - Sodium bicarbonate can be used.
  - Avoid diuretics, which may further exacerbate hypotension and electrolyte abnormalities.
  - Renal-replacement therapy (RRT), including hemodialysis. CVVH may be required in severe cases.

Contrast-Induced Nephropathy

➤ **Definition:**

Nephrotoxicity caused by administration of iodinated contrast agent for diagnostic purposes. The majority of the contrast agents currently in use are iodine based. The most commonly used contrast mediums currently in use have the potential to cause renal impairment by 25%. Majority of these contrast agents are used in radiology (CT, MRI), and cardiology (cardiac catheterization) The degree of nephrotoxicity could range from a mild deterioration of kidney function to acute renal failure.

➤ **Pathophysiology:**

Renal blood flow is diminished due to vasoconstriction of the medullary blood vessels. Reduced blood flow results in lower oxygen concentration in the renal parenchyma, which makes the medulla susceptible to the injurious effects of the contrast medium. This results in ischemic necrosis of the renal tubules. Cytokines and other oxygen-based free radicals are released as the ischemic necrosis ensues, causing havoc and exacerbating the injurious process.

➤ **Risk Factors:**

- Dehydration
- Underlying kidney failure
- Diabetes mellitus
- Types and amount of contrast given
- Low perfusion status, i.e., CHF, cirrhosis

➤ **Prevention/Treatment:**

- Analyze benefit versus risk ratio in patients undergoing diagnostic studies or procedures that require IV contrast administration.
- Optimize underlying medical condition, diabetes mellitus, kidney failure, or congestive heart failure prior to the contrast administration.
- Stop all potential nephrotoxic agents, i.e., metformin, NSAIDs.

- Hydration prior to during and after dye is given seems to ameliorate the sequalae of contrast-induced nephropathy.
- Bicarbonate-containing solutions can also be given in some cases.
- N-acetylcysteine (NAC or Mucomyst) was previously a popular antioxidant agent for the prevention of contrast-induced nephropathy. Recent studies, however, did not corroborate the benefit that it once promised for preventing contrast-induced nephropathy.

Surgical, Trauma and Procedural Emergencies

1. Abdominal Compartment Syndrome
2. Extremity Compartment Syndrome
3. Complications of Nasogastric and Orogastric (NG/OG) Tube
4. Posterior Pharyngeal Perforation
5. Air Embolism
6. Shock
7. Burn Management
8. Blast Injuries
9. Crush Injuries

Abdominal Compartment Syndrome (ACS)

> Definition:

The terms intra-abdominal hypertension (IAH) and ACS are used interchangeably in literature.

This clinical syndrome is characterized by:

- Increased intra-abdominal pressure >20-25 mmHg
- Resultant organ dysfunction
  - **Respiratory failure:** Patients will often require ventilator support. However, if the patient is already on the ventilator, it becomes extremely difficult to ventilate as a result of the increasing abdominal pressure and resultant stress on the diaphragm and the respiratory

system. All ventilator-related pressures may go up, i.e., PIP (peak inspiratory pressure), Pplat (plateau pressure).

- **Cardiac dysfunction:** Hemodynamic compromise resulting in shock, which often requires vasopressor support. This occurs due to compression of the inferior vena cava and decreased venous return.
- **Renal failure:** ACS may result in decreased urinary output and acute renal failure. This is due to the compromised vascular supply to the renal tubules.

➤ **Risk Factors:**
  - Trauma
  - Recent abdominal surgery
  - Critical illness

➤ **Mechanisms:**
  - Increased retroperitoneal volume (edema from pancreatitis, hemorrhage from pelvic trauma or post aortic injury)
  - Increase intraperitoneal volume (hemorrhage, bowel distension, mesenteric venous obstruction, tense ascites, or abdominal packing)
  - Extrinsic compression (burns, eschar, tight abdominal closure)

➤ **Diagnosis:**
  - Urinary bladder pressure monitoring
  - Diagnosis is made on clinical grounds

➤ **How to measure intra-abdominal pressures:**
  - **Direct method:** By placing intraperitoneal catheter
  - **Indirect method:** By measuring the abdominal pressure through the urinary bladder (Foley's catheter). Inject 60cc of sterile saline into the bladder, while the distal aspiration port is clamped. The pressure transducer apparatus is then hooked up to the aspiration port of the Foley's catheter. The pressure can be measured through the CVP transducer.

➤ **Treatment:**
- Mechanical ventilatory support may be necessary if the patient is not already intubated.
- Patient may have to be paralyzed to reduce the intra-abdominal pressure and support ventilation.
- Immediate consultation by a surgeon may be required to evaluate surgical candidacy of the patient. If surgery is performed, the abdomen is often left open, using a Bogota bag (Balad bag—used during Iraq war) with secondary closure within 48 hours.

Extremity Compartment Syndrome
Usually manifests in the upper or lower extremities

➤ **Etiology:**
- Long bone fracture—tibia and forearm are the most commonly involved bones
- Snake bite
- Trauma
- Casts and tight compressive bandages
- Burns/eschar
- Post limb surgery
- Pressure ulcers caused by prolonged immobilization
- Spontaneous extremity syndrome may occur in the lower extremities, especially during long marathon run

➤ **Clinical Features (6 Ps):**
- Pallor
- Pain (usually a late phenomenon)
- Pulseless
- Paresthesia
- Paralysis (usually an irreversible damage at this point)
- Progression of symptoms

➤ **Diagnosis:**
- Diagnosis is made on clinical grounds

- Can be confirmed by measuring compartment pressure invasively
➤ **How to Measure Extremity Pressure (materials needed):**
  - Intra-compartment needle (18-gauge needle with side-port)
  - High-pressure tubing (like the arterial line set)
  - Pressure transducer with a cable
  - Pressure monitor
  - Sterile saline
  - Transducer stand
  - Two 3-way stopcocks
  - Syringe, 20 mL
➤ **Preparation and the Procedure:**
  - Prepare the skin in a sterile fashion
  - Use topical lidocaine or any local anesthetic to achieve the numbing effect
  - Moderate sedation can be used in agitated or uncooperative patients
  - Patient can be positioned supine or prone
  - The compartment measured should be at the heart level—"Zero"
  - Remove tourniquets
  - The lower leg has four compartments: anterior, lateral, deep posterior, and superficial posterior. The anterior lower leg is the most commonly affected compartment. The needle should be placed three cm on either side of a transverse line drawn at the junction of the proximal and middle thirds of the lower leg. The needle placement should be confirmed by a several-fold increase in the pressure tracing upon dorsiflexion or plantar flexion of the foot.
➤ **Treatment:**
  - Fasciatomy
  - Escharatomy (in case of burns)

Complications of NG/OT Tube

Nasogastric/orogastric tubes can be inadvertently placed in the lung, especially in patients with compromised gag, cough reflex, and altered mental status. The following complications may occur:

- Pneumothorax
- Atelectasis
- Pleural effusion
- Bronchopleural fistula
- Hydrothorax
- Empyema
- Pneumonitis
- Oropharyngeal perforation
- Epistaxis (nosebleed)
- Downed lung (complete or near complete opacification of one lung)
  - CXR — worsening infiltrate/pleural effusion
  - Usually one lung is affected

Posterior Pharyngeal Perforation

➢ **Definition:**
- Loss of integrity of the posterior pharyngeal soft tissue/ membrane, caused by iatrogenic trauma. Can be caused by intubation, EGD, TEE, or bronchoscopy (rigid>flexible).

➢ **Signs/Symptoms:**
- Fever
- Neck pain
- Dysphagia
- Hoarseness
- Tenderness

➢ **Etiology:**
- Instrumentation (bronchoscopy, flexible or rigid), esophagogastroduodenoscopy (EGD), laryngoscopy, transesophageal echocardiography (TEE), endotracheal/ nasotracheal (ET/NT) intubation, or nasogastric/orogastric

tube insertion

> **Risk factors:**
  - Congenital abnormalities, i.e., cleft palate
  - Burns due to friable tissue
  - Chemical ingestion of a strong alkali, i.e., lye or acids such as sulphuric acid
  - Recent radiation/chemotherapy, which renders the membranes of the soft tissue quite friable, making them susceptible to damage
  - Recent ear, nose, or throat (FNT) surgery
> **Diagnosis:**
  - Chest x-ray shows subcutaneous air
  - Confirmatory test—barium esophogram
> **Treatment:**
  - Nonsurgical
    - Endoscopic irrigation
    - Fibrin glue
    - Endoscopic clipping
  - Surgical
    - <12 hours — primary closure and drainage
    - >12 hours — drainage only

Air Embolism

> **Definition:**
  - Air entry from atmosphere into the systemic circulation
> **Etiology:**
  - Central venous access/PICC line placement
  - PA catheter/pacemaker insertion
  - Pregnancy
  - Surgery
  - Barotrauma
> **Clinical:**
  - Obstruction of right-sided outflow
  - Hemodynamic compromise, hypotension

- Paradoxical emboli, with pre-existing ASD/VSD
- 300-500 mL of air in the circulation can be fatal

➢ **Diagnosis:**
- Clinical setting (iatrogenic)
- Sudden hemodynamic collapse or syncope
- CT scan of the chest
- Echocardiogram, may show air bubbles
- "Washing machine murmur" on physical exam

➢ **Complications:**
- Cerebrovascular accident/transient ischemic attacks (CVA/TIA)
- Seizures
- Coma, persistent vegetative state, and death

➢ **Treatment:**
- Lateral decubitus position
- Trendelenburg position
- High flow and high fractional oxygen (100% FiO2)
- Hyperbaric chamber, if available
- Manual removal of the air by inserting a catheter in the major vein and right atrium, if recent embolization

Shock

➢ **Definition:**
- Circulatory failure that causes tissue hypoperfusion and hypoxia

➢ **Types of Shock:**
- Hemorrhagic (trauma or bleeding/clotting disorders)
  - Class I: up to 15% blood loss or less than 750 ml
  - Class II: 15-30% blood loss or 750-1500 ml
  - Class III: 30-40% blood loss or 1500-2000 ml
  - Class IV: >40% blood loss or greater than 2000 ml
- Hypovolemic (dehydration, diarrhea, vomiting, heat stroke)
- Cardiogenic (myocardial infarction)

- Tension pneumothorax (surgical/medical emergency)
- Neurogenic (head and neck or spinal cord injury)
- Obstructive (pulmonary embolism, cardiac tamponade)
- Distributive (sepsis, burns)

➢ **Signs/Symptoms:**
- Circulatory failure, hypotension, tachycardia
- Neurogenic shock is an exception; it presents with hypotension and relative bradycardia. This type of shock usually doesn't improve with volume resuscitation.

➢ **Terrible Triad:**
- Hypothermia
- Acidosis
- Coagulopathy

➢ **Treatment:**
- Volume resuscitation with blood, normal saline, Ringer's lactate (LR)
- Cover the patient with warm blankets to prevent hypothermia
- Warm all fluids, i.e., saline, Ringer's lactate, and blood products
- Rapid transfuser with warmer should be used. Blood products can't be microwaved.
- Whole blood should be used, if available, during the hemorrhagic shock. If fractionated blood products are used, a transfusion strategy of 1:1:1 should be employed. This entails one unit of PRBC, followed by one unit of platelet and one unit of albumin. Cryoprecipitate should be transfused after a few units of FFP.
- Occasionally calcium supplementation may be necessary when massive transfusion is given (more than 10 units of PRBC). Stored blood is often citrated to prolong its shelf-life. It can also precipitate further depleting the calcium concentration in the blood.
- Adverse events—i.e., ABO mismatch, anaphylaxis, TACO,

- and TRALI—should be duly recognized and promptly treated.
- Definite treatment strategy rests on early diagnosis and treatment of the underlying cause of the shock.

Burns Management Principles

➤ **Definition:**

Multitude of tissue and organ injuries sustained by toxic effects of fumes, chemical and thermal sources

➤ **Types of Burns:**

- **First-Degree Burns**

  Superficial burns sustained as a result of mild burns. The most common example of the first-degree burn is sunburn, which is characterized by damage to the epidermis. Clinically presents as erythema and blistering of the skin. This kind of burn is often painful in nature, due to injury and exposure of the nerve endings. Usually heals within a few days.

- **Second-Degree Burns**

  The burn runs deeper than the superficial burns and involves the dermis in addition to the epidermis. Second-degree burn may present similar to the first-degree burn, i.e., skin blistering and local pain. The healing process is prolonged, and may take a few weeks as compared with first-degree burns.

- **Third-Degree Burns**

  These are full thickness burns that reach the deep tissues and structures. The appearance of skin may be leathery. Pain is often absent due to destruction of the nerve endings, which are present in the superficial skin layers such as the dermis and epidermis.

- **Fourth-Degree Burns**

  These kinds of burns involve muscles and tendons. They appear charred and black in appearance and again are not very painful, since nerve endings are destroyed.

➤ **Estimation of the Surface Area Affected by Burns**
- Rules of Nine
- Lund and Browder nomogram

➤ **Burn Management:**
- The most critical part in the initial management of the burn victim is to accurately determine the body surface area burnt; calculation is made according to the percentage of second- and third-degree burns.
- IV access, at least two large bore vascular lines, preferably 16 gauge, should be placed.
- Central line, if can be placed within reasonable amount of time, as resuscitation should not be delayed due to the lack of the central venous access
- Mechanical ventilation and early intubation, if inhalational injury is evident or suspected. The typical signs of inhalational or airway injury are singed facial hair, soot around the nose or mouth, and any carbonaceous sputum.
- Use vasopressors if the patient is hypotensive. This is initiated early to avoid further tissue damage due to organ hypoperfusion.
- Hydrocortisone for relative adrenal insufficiency, especially when patient is hypotensive in spite of ongoing or optimal fluid resuscitation and vasopressor support
- Local wound care
- Tetanus prophylaxis, if indicated
- Prophylactic antibiotics, if sepsis is a concern
- Topical antimicrobials, i.e., silver sulfadiazine
- Escharatomy for the extremity or circumferential torso burns
- Corrective surgery, i.e., fasciatomy for the extremity burns with compartment syndrome
- Laparotomy if abdominal compartment syndrome
- Management of shock

- Fluid resuscitation, multiple formulas are used;
  - □ Parkland Formula
  - □ Brooks Formula
  - □ Warden Formula
- ➤ Half of the calculated fluid is given in the first eight hours, and the rest is administered over the next 16 hours. LR is often preferred, and warm solution should be given to prevent hypothermia especially with associated shock. The initial fluid resuscitation given in the field is also taken into account when calculating the total amount of fluid to be administered. The required resuscitation fluid amount should be calculated from the initial injury rather than after arrival in the ER or ICU. Conventional methods of resuscitation, Parkland Formula tend to over-resuscitate. This approach may be detrimental due to worsening clinical outcomes. Therefore, a rather conservative approach should be utilized in the initial resuscitative efforts. Bedside clinical judgment should be paramount in the initial burn management as individual clinical case scenarios may pose challenges where an individualized versus protocolized approach should be used. These formulas should be used as guidelines rather than rules. Resuscitation should be guided by clinical outcomes such as blood pressure, heart rate, and urine output. Albumin can also be used, especially during the maintenance phase, which follows the initial twenty-four hours of fluid resuscitation.
- ➤ **Under-resuscitation**
  - Low urine output and renal failure
  - Low blood pressure and hemodynamic instability
  - Shock and acidosis
- ➤ **Over-resuscitation**
  - Fluid overload and respiratory failure
  - Compartment syndromes, abdominal or extremity
  - Third spacing, which occurs due to the escape of fluid from the intravascular space to the extracellular space and is exacerbated by the capillary leak and low oncotic pressure

Blast Injuries

➢ **Definition:**

Multitude of tissue and organ injuries sustained by blasts

➢ **Agents Causing Blast Injuries:**

- **High-Order Blast Agents**
  - Nitroglycerine
  - Dynamite
  - Plastique
  - Ammonium nitrate
  - Trinitrotoluene (TNT)
- **Low-Order Blast Agents**
  - Petroleum products; "Molotov Cocktail"
  - Gunpowder
  - Pipe bomb
- **Secondary Agents**
  - Shrapnel
  - Contaminants that may be biological or environmental

➢ **Types of Blast Injuries:**

- **Primary Blast Injuries**
  - Pressure injury caused by the blast wave
  - Rupture of the tympanic membrane (eardrum); most common blast injury
  - Blast lung-pulmonary contusion
  - Traumatic brain injury (TBI)
  - Hollow viscus; abdominal organ injury
- **Secondary Blast Injuries**
  - Injuries caused by penetrating wounds from flying debris, shrapnel, and foreign objects
  - Head and neck and bony fractures account for most of the injuries
- **Tertiary Blast Injuries**
  - Caused by the blast wind
  - Skull, bones, and head and neck injuries
  - Crush injuries

- **Quaternary Blast Injuries**
  - Other factors causing the injury such as radiation or heat
  - Burns
  - Exacerbation of an underlying medical condition, asthma, COPD
  - Rhabdomyolysis
- ➢ **Pathophysiology:**
  - Rapid conversions of solid or liquid into gaseous form
  - Compression of the atmospheric gases due to rapid gas expansion
  - Pressure wave and wind created by this effect spread in all directions
  - The injury pattern varies depending on the environment in which blast occurred, open versus closed spaces
  - Injury occurs by;
    - **Spalling**—Disruption of the tissues because of the blast wave
    - **Implosion**—Hollow organ injury due to the expansion of pre-existing gases
    - **Shearing Forces**—Tissue tearing
- ➢ **Clinical Presentation:**
  - Most of the patients (75%) are ambulatory upon initial presentation
  - The presentation depends on multiple factors:
    - Organs involved
    - Open or closed blast environment
    - Distance from the blast
- ➢ **Treatment:**
  - Appropriate triage
  - Oxygen/ventilatory support/intubation
  - Hemodynamic support, fluid, vasopressors
  - Look and treat, rhabdomyolysis, extremity and abdominal compartment syndrome

X-RAY SKULL AP VIEW (FOREIGN BODY IN THE HEAD)

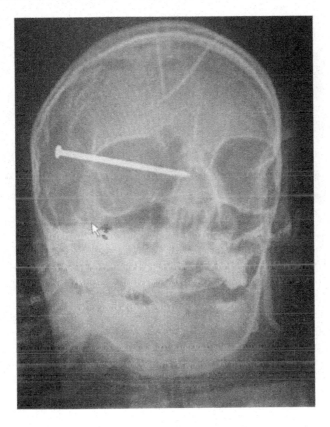

X-RAY SKULL AP VIEW (FOREIGN BODY IN THE HEAD)

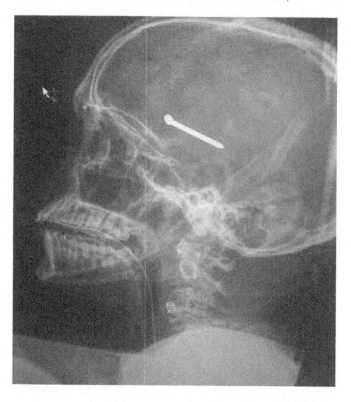

Crush Injuries

➤ **Definition:**

Injuries sustained when subjected to high degree or prolonged exposure to force or pressure. These injuries result from traumatic or non-traumatic causes: direct muscle damage, toxin-mediated injury, rhabdomyolysis, and the effects of medications.

➤ **Type of Injuries:**

- Extremity compartment syndrome
- Reperfusion injuries

➤ **Causes:**

- Natural disasters, tornados, earthquakes, or hurricanes
- Building or structural collapse
- Motor vehicle accident (MVA)
- Prolonged immobilization
- Blast injuries

➤ **Clinical Outcomes:**

- Electrolyte abnormalities
- Renal failure
- Arrhythmias
- Disseminated intravascular coagulation (DIC)
- Acidosis

➤ **Treatment:**

- Early recognition (Use ATLS protocol-ABCD)
- Supportive care
- Ventilatory support
- Hemodynamic support
- Electrolyte replacement
- Assess for hemodialysis need
- Pain control
- Shock treatment

Endocrine Considerations in the ICU

1. Thyroid Storm
2. Euthyroid Sick Syndrome
3. Serotonin Syndrome
4. Drugs Associated with Serotonin Syndrome
5. Myxedema Coma
6. Fat Embolism Syndrome
7. Diabetic Ketoacidosis (DKA)
8. Hyperosmolar Non-Ketotic State (HONK) or Hyperosmolar Hyperglycemic State (HHS)

Thyroid Storm

➢ **Definition:** Occurs in patients with history of inadequately treated Graves' disease, leading to thyrotoxicosis. This can be caused a host of factors, including:
  ▪ Surgery
  ▪ Infection
  ▪ Exogenous thyroid supplementation
  ▪ Toxic goiter
  ▪ Thyroiditis
  ▪ Thyroid adenoma
  ▪ Thyroid cancer
➢ **Clinical symptoms** (due to catecholamine excess):
  ▪ Tachycardia/tachyarrhythmia
  ▪ Delirium and psychosis

- Hyperpyrexia
- Hypertension (HTN)
- Hyperreflexia
- High output congestive heart failure (CHF)

➤ **Laboratory Findings:**
  - Decreased TSH (high serum levels send a negative feedback response)
  - Increased T3/T4 (active hormones)

➤ **Treatment:**

Beta blockade is the cornerstone treatment modality for the thyroid storm. Nonspecific beta-blockers, i.e., propranolol, are the best initial therapy because they block both alpha- and beta-receptors. This is followed by the administration of propylthiouracil (PTU). This blocks peripheral conversion of T4 to T3, thus reducing the serum concentration of the metabolically active hormones. Lugol solution or potassium iodide can be given one hour after PTU and steroids. Intravenous route should be used for the administration of these medicines in the acute setting.

Euthyroid Sick Syndrome

➤ **Definition:** Lab abnormalities suggest pituitary or thyroid dysfunction

➤ **Laboratory Findings:**
  - Thyroid-stimulating hormone (TSH) normal or low
  - Decreased T3, T4
  - Increased (reverse-T3) rT3

➤ **Pathogenesis:**
  - Decreased conversion of T4 to T3
  - Impaired rT3 clearance
  - Adaptive response to conserve energy especially during any critical illness

➤ **Predisposing factors:**
  - Sepsis

- Burn
- Malignancy
- Myocardial infarction (MI)
- Trauma/surgery
➢ **Treatment:**
  - Observation; provide supportive care
➢ **Differential Diagnosis:**
  - Secondary hypothyroidism
  - Pituitary causes
  - Hypothalamic causes

* Routine testing of the thyroid function is not suggested, especially during times of stress, as the lab values may not be reflective of the true hormonal status. This may lead to unnecessary diagnostic work-up, treatment, or delays in life-saving procedures, i.e., surgery. Thyroid testing should only be performed when there are symptoms or clinical indications suggestive of abnormal functional thyroid status.

Serotonin Syndrome

➢ **Definition:** Potentially life-threatening condition caused by too much serotonin release in the central nervous system
➢ **Signs/symptoms:**
  - Altered mental status
  - Neuromuscular hyperactivity/hyperexcitability
    □ Hyperreflexia
    □ Clonus
    □ Muscular rigidity
  - Autonomic hyperactivity (agitation, tremors, diaphoresis, mydriasis, dry oral mucosa, hypertension, and tachycardia)
  - Extreme cases:
  Temperature elevation (hyperthermia), shock, acidosis, rhabdomyolysis, acute renal failure (ARF), and respiratory failure

➤ **Treatment:**
  - Supportive
  - Severe hyperthermia: intubate and paralyze with neuro-muscular blocking agent
  - Benzodiazepines for muscle relaxation
  - Dantrolene

➤ **Differential Diagnosis:**
  - Neuroleptic malignant syndrome
  - Anticholinergic syndrome
  - Malignant hyperthermia
  - Acute lithium toxicity

Drugs Associated With Serotonin Syndrome:

➤ **Antidepressants**
  - Selective serotonin reuptake inhibitor (SSRI)
  - Monoamine oxidase inhibitor (MAOI)
  - Tricyclic antidepressants TCA (trazadone, buspirone)

➤ **Anticonvulsants** (valproate)

➤ **Analgesics** (merperidine, fentanyl, tramadol)

➤ **Antiemetic** (ondansetron, metoclopramide)

➤ **Anti-migraine** (sumatriptan)

➤ **Antibiotics** (linezolid, rifaximin)

➤ **Antitussive** (dextromethorphan)

➤ **Bariatric** (sibutramine)

➤ **Drugs of abuse** (ecstasy, LSD, cocaine)

➤ **Dietary supplements** (ginseng, tryptophan, St. John's Wort)

➤ **Neuropsychiatric** (lithium)

Myxedema Coma

➤ **Definition:** Extreme and potentially life-threatening condition, caused by decreased levels of active thyroid hormones, i.e., T3, T4

➤ **Clinical:**
  - Lethargy, which may present as alteration of mental status

or coma
- Adynamic or paralytic ileus due to gut hypomotility
- Hypothermia
- Hypercarbic respiratory failure
- Slow atrial fibrillation
- Slow deep tendon reflex (DTR) relaxation
- Congestive heart failure (CHF)

➢ **Laboratory Findings:**
- Increased TSH (low serum levels send a positive feedback)
- Decreased T3 and T4 (low levels of active hormones)

➢ **Treatment:**
- Intravenous thyroxin (T4)
- Hydrocortisone should be given concurrently until adrenal insufficiency is ruled out or corrected. This can be determined by a quick assessment of the random serum cortisol level.

Fat Embolism Syndrome

➢ **Definition:**
A symptom complex of neurologic dysfunction associated with hypoxia. It is caused by absorption and embolization of fat globules after long bony fracture due to trauma or orthopedic manipulation.

➢ **Signs/symptoms:**
- Hypoxia
- Diffuse pulmonary infiltrate
- Confusion and altered mental status
- Petechial rash, most common on the anterior chest wall or upper torso
- Fever
- Thrombocytopenia
- Oliguria

➢ **Risk factors:**
- Long bone fracture
- Post orthopedics procedure

- Liposuction
- Sickle cell crisis
- Tumor lysis syndrome (TLS), post induction chemotherapy, especially in hematopoietic cancers, i.e., leukemia, lymphoma
- Pancreatitis
- Lipid infusion (TPN)

➤ **Prevention:**
  - Orthopedic surgery: Use of special orthopedic procedures that minimize the risk of fat embolism
  - Early fracture stabilization prior to surgery

➤ **Treatment:**
  - Supportive care
  - Steroids: IV methylprednisolone 1.5 mg/kg Q8H x 6 dose

Diabetic Ketoacidosis (DKA)

➤ **Definition:**
Extreme metabolic derangement caused by excessive acid accumulation in the blood. This catabolic process results from the absence or deficiency of insulin. DKA is often seen in patients with Type-1 diabetes mellitus.

➤ **Pathophysiology:**
  - Acids build up in the serum due to utilization of the free fatty acids, which are used in lieu of carbohydrates in the insulin deficient environment.
  - There are three types of endogenous ketone bodies, which are formed as a result of fat breakdown. The presence of these ketones causes the pH to decrease and results in acidosis. The acetone breath or the fruity odor in the DKA patient is caused by the presence of these fatty acid breakdown products:
    - Acetone (volatile gas)
    - Acetoacetic acid
    - Beta-hydroxybutric acid

> **Signs/symptoms:**
  - Excessive thirst and dehydration
  - Polyuria
  - Nausea, vomiting and abdominal pain (most common)
  - Anorexia
  - Weakness
  - Shortness of breath
  - Altered mental status, confusion, and coma
> **Diagnosis:**
  - Clinical presentation and history of DM (DKA may be the initial presentation of DM)
  - High serum glucose level (usually in the 500 range, but DKA can also occur with relatively low blood glucose levels)
  - Increased serum and urine osmolality
  - Ketones in the blood and urine
  - Electrolyte imbalances
  - Signs and symptoms of dehydration
  - CBC, CMP, CXR, urinalysis, or other tests to look for the source of infection
  - EKG
> **Differential Diagnosis:**
  - Alcoholism can cause ketosis
  - Fasting or starvation ketoacidosis
> **Risk Factors:**
  - Type-I DM
  - Uncontrolled glycemic index (elevated HbA1C)
  - History of noncompliance
  - Stressors such as infection, surgery, and trauma
> **Preventions:**
  - Tight glucose control
  - Preventive measures such as good foot care (podiatrist visits once a year) and administration of flu and pneumonia vaccinations

➤ **Treatment:**
  - Insulin infusion till the AG is closed <12
  - Fluid resuscitation
  - Electrolyte replacements
  - Control and treatment of infection
  - Oxygen or ventilatory support
  - Supportive measure

Hyperosmolar Non-Ketotic State (HONK) or Hyperosmolar Hyperglycemic State (HHS)

➤ **Definition:**
  Extreme elevation of the serum glucose levels above 500 mg/dl, usually in the 1000 range. It is associated with little or no acid accumulation, which is a hallmark of DKA. This condition is often seen in patients with Type-II diabetes mellitus. There is severe dehydration associated with this state, which results in very high plasma osmolality.

➤ **Pathophysiology:**
  The severe dehydration is caused by osmotic diuresis due to very high serum osmolality. This in turn results in cellular dehydration in conjunction with the osmotic diuresis.

  Signs/symptoms:
  - Excessive thirst and dehydration
  - Altered mental status, confusion, coma (more common than DKA)
  - Polyuria
  - Nausea, vomiting and abdominal pain (less common)
  - Anorexia
  - Weakness
  - Shortness of breath

➤ **Diagnosis:**
  - Clinical presentation
  - High serum glucose level often in the thousand range (higher than DKA)

- Increased serum and urine osmolality
- Little or no ketones in the blood and urine
- Electrolyte imbalances
- Signs and symptoms of dehydration
- CBC, CMP, CXR, urinalysis, or other tests to look for the source of infection
- EKG
- ➢ **Risk factors:**
  - Type-II DM
  - Uncontrolled glycemic index (HbA-1C)
  - History of noncompliance
  - Stressors such as infections, surgery, and trauma
- ➢ **Preventions:**
  - Tight glucose control
  - Preventive medicine principles similar to DKA
- ➢ **Treatment:**
  - Insulin infusion
  - Aggressive fluid resuscitation
    - *Rapid correction of the AG or lowering of the serum glucose levels (both in DKA and HHS treatment) should be avoided to prevent catastrophic events, i.e., central pontine myelonolysis (CPM).*

Critical Care Toxicology

1. Compounds That Can Be Removed by Hemodialysis (HD)
2. Tricyclic Antidepressant (TCA) Overdose
3. Drugs Causing Prolonged QT
4. Propofol-Related Infusion Syndrome (PRIS)
5. Alcohol Intoxication
6. Propylene Glycol Toxicity
7. Ethylene Glycol Toxicity
8. Gamma Hydroxybutyrate (GHB) or "Date Rape Drug"
9. Serotonin Syndrome
10. Malignant Hyperthermia
11. Carbon Monoxide (CO) Poisoning
12. Stevens-Johnson Syndrome (SJS) & Toxic Epidermal Necrolysis (TEN)
13. Lidocaine Toxicity
14. Calcium Channel Blockers (CCB) Toxicity
15. Beta-Blockers (BB) Toxicity

Compounds That Can Be Removed by Hemodialysis:

- Ethylene glycol
- Methanol
- Salicylate
- Theophylline
- Lithium
- Vancomycin

Not Dialyzable Compounds
Selective Serotonin Reuptake Inhibitor (SSRI)

Tricyclic Antidepressant (TCA) Overdose
➢ **Major Effects:**
- **Central adrenergic blockade**
  - Coma
  - Hypotension
  - Seizure
- **Antiarrhythmic properties**
  - QRS prolongation/QT prolongation
  - Arrhythmia
- **Anticholinergic properties**
  - Tachycardia
  - Hyperthermia
  - Dry mucous membranes
  - Mydriasis
  - Decreased GI motility
  - Urinary retention

➢ **Treatment:**
- Charcoal
- Bicarbonate with goal to keep serum pH 7.5-755
- Norepinephrine may be indicated for hypotension
- Gastric lavage may be done early in the course of ingestion
- Physostigmine can be used in refractory TCA overdose, but also causes arrhythmia

Drugs Causing Prolonged QT
➢ **Neuro and Psychotropic Drugs:**
- Methadone
- Haldol
- Tricyclic Antidepressants (TCA)

➢ **Cardiac Drugs:**
- Amiodarone

- Quinolone
- Digoxin
- Antiarrhythmic
  - Sotalol
  - Ibutilide
  - Procainamide
  - Disopyramide
➤ **Antimicrobial:**
- Antifungals
- Macrolides
- Quinine
  * Vancomycin DOES NOT cause prolonged QT

Propofol-Related Infusion Syndrome (PRIS)

➤ **Definition:**

It is a clinical condition characterized by a profound electrolyte imbalance and associated hemodynamic instability. This is caused by high dose and prolonged propofol infusion. This can potentially lead to multiple organ failure or death.

➤ **Risk Factors:**
- Fatal condition (most commonly in the pediatric population)
- Long-term infusions (>48h)
- When doses exceed >5 mg/kg/hr

➤ **Clinical:**
- Severe metabolic acidosis
- Rhabdomyolysis
- Hyperkalemia
- Renal failure
- Heart failure
- Arrhythmia

➤ **Pathogenesis:**
- Uncoupling of oxidative phosphorylation in mitochondria
- Impaired fatty acid oxidation
- Excess catecholamine release

➢ **Treatment:**
- ▪ Stop propofol
- ▪ Supportive care

Alcohol Intoxication

➢ **Diagnosis:**

● **Step-I**

First check osmolar gap (measured plasma osmolality minus the calculated osmolality) >20 is abnormal

Ethanol, methanol, ethylene glycol, and isopropyl alcohols can increase osmolality

● **Step-II**

Check anion gap
- ▪ Increased gap seen in methanol and ethylene glycol
- ▪ No anion gap is seen with isopropyl, acetone, and ketonuria

  * Isopropyl ("iso" means same) can be correlated with the AG, which also remains the same.

➢ **Treatment:**
- ▪ Methanol, ethylene glycol produce toxic metabolites.
- ▪ Ethanol and fomepizole inhibits formation of these metabolites.
- ▪ Isopropyl alcohol becomes acetone since there is no inhibition. Hemodialysis may be needed for a level greater than 400 mg/dL.
- ▪ Methanol can cause permanent blindness, and therefore early ophthalmology consult is indicated.
- ▪ Bicarbonate infusion may be indicated to prevent crystallization and precipitation of the metabolites in the renal tubules. The ethylene glycol forms uric acid crystals, which may precipitate in the urine. These crystals can be visualized under microscopy as envelope-shaped crystals; hence bicarbonate infusion will prevent acute tubular necrosis (ATN) and resultant renal failure.

Propylene Glycol Toxicity

- ➤ Presents with metabolic acidosis
- ➤ Osmolar gap
- ➤ **Etiologic agents** (agents in ethylene glycol):
  - Lorazepam
  - Diazepam
  - Topical silver sulfadiazine
  - IV nitroglycerin
  - Etomidate
  - Phenytoin
- ➤ **Clinical:**
  - Hyperosmolarity
  - Hemolytic anemia
  - Arrhythmia
  - Seizures
  - Coma
  - Lactic acidosis
  - Hypertension
- ➤ **Metabolism:**
  - 45% excreted by kidney
  - 55% metabolized by liver, with the byproducts:
    - □ Lactic acid
    - □ Pyruvic acid
    - □ Acetone
- ➤ **Treatment:**
  - □ Stop infusion of the suspect medication

Ethylene Glycol Toxicity

Found in antifreeze, brake fluid, industrial solvent

- ➤ Poisoning—lethal dose 1.4 ml/kg
- ➤ **Clinical**: Inebriation similar to alcohol intoxication
  - **30 minutes-12 hours (CNS)**
  - Confusion
  - Somnolence

- Agitation
- **12-24 hours (fatal stage)**
- Worsening of neurological status
- Heart failure
- Respiratory failure
- **24-72 hours (renal failure)**

➤ **Laboratory Findings:**
  - Anion gap (AG) metabolic acidosis from both glycolic and lactic acids
  - Increased osmolar gap
  - Calcium oxalate crystals formation
  - AG appears later than the osmolar gap because of the longer time for glycolic acid formation
  - Hypocalcaemia due to precipitation of calcium oxalate crystals
  - Negative assay for methanol

➤ **Treatment:**
  - Should be started promptly
  - Fomepizole given intravenously acts as an antidote by competitively inhibiting alcohol dehydrogenase
  - Loading dose: 15 mg/kg, followed by 10 mg/kg q12h x 4 doses, then 15 mg/kg q12h thereafter until ethylene glycol levels <20 mg/dl
  - Hemodialysis
    It should be considered in addition to the fomepizole when there are any of the following situations:
    - Severe acidosis (refractory to bicarbonate)
    - Renal failure
    - Hemodynamic instability
  - Thiamine/pyridoxine—counteracts toxins
  - Hydration
  - NG lavage within the first hour of ingestion and ER presentation
  - Avoid calcium supplementation

- The dose of fomepizole should be given every four hours
- It is dialyzable

➤ **Pathogenesis:**
- Ethylene glycol is metabolized in the liver by alcohol dehydrogenase to:
  - Glycolic acid
  - Oxalic acid

Gamma Hydroxybutyrate (GHB) "Date Rape Drug"

➤ **Gamma Hydroxybutyric Acid**
Colorless, odorless liquid that is very easy to add to any drink

➤ **Reasons for Abuse:**
- Rape
- Euphoria
- Memory loss
- Sleep/drowsiness
- Anabolic agent in body builders
- Increased libido

➤ **Higher Doses:**
- Respiratory depression
- Coma
- Seizure
- Bradycardia
- Hypothermia

➤ **Antidote:**
None available; therefore, provide supportive measures

➤ **Recovery:**
- Rapid
- Extubation comes quickly if patient requires intubation
  - *Dispensed through the central pharmacy in the USA to prevent abuse of the drug*

Serotonin Syndrome

Syndrome characterized by a surge of "brain hormone" serotonin in blood, which is essentially similar to "catecholamine rush." Serotonin syndrome most often occurs when two drugs that affect the body's level of serotonin are taken together. Occasional overdose of serotonergic medication may cause this syndrome.

> ➢ **Symptoms** occur within minutes to hours, and may include:
>   - Agitation or restlessness
>   - Diarrhea
>   - Fast heartbeat
>   - Hallucinations
>   - Increased body temperature
>   - Loss of coordination
>   - Nausea
>   - Overactive reflexes
>   - Rapid changes in blood pressure
>   - Vomiting
>   □ *Causes systemic effects such as hyperthermia, hypertension, and muscle rigidity*
>   □ *Frequently seen in drug overdose or after coming out of anesthesia*

Malignant Hyperthermia

Malignant hyperthermia is a disease passed down through families that causes a rapid increase in body temperature and severe muscle contractions when the affected person receives general anesthesia.

> ➢ **Symptoms:**
>   - Bleeding
>   - Dark brown urine
>   - Muscle ache without an obvious cause such as exercise or injury
>   - Muscle rigidity and stiffness
>   - Quick rise in body temperature to 105 degrees F or higher
>   - Malignant hyperthermia is often discovered after a patient

is given anesthesia during surgery
- There may be family history of malignant hyperthermia or unexplained death during anesthesia
- The person may have a fast and irregular heartbeat

➢ **Treatment:**

Supportive care: oxygen, intubation, Ativan, deep sedation

Treat early to prevent seizures and brain damage

Carbon Monoxide (CO) Poisoning OR "Invisible or Quiet Killer"

➢ **Definition:**

Carbon monoxide causes a sudden and often lethal poisoning. This is often accidental or suicidal in nature due to its characteristic of being an odorless, colorless, and hence toxic gas. It is found in common combustible sources such as motor vehicles, gas engines, heating systems, and gas cooking ranges. It is a common byproduct of the fumes emanating from cigarette smoke and results in the sequalae of secondhand smoke. Higher levels of carbon monoxide are often detected in non-smoking urban dwellers without any clinical consequence.

➢ **Etiology:**

Inhalation of the fumes under conditions when there is absence of fresh air or lack of proper ventilation. This results in the recirculation of the gas in the confined space, causing toxicity.

- Accidental
- Suicidal
- Homicidal

➢ **Types of Poisoning Based on Exposure:**

- Acute
- Chronic

➢ **Signs and Symptoms:**

- Confusion
- Lethargy
- Disorientation

- Nausea/vomiting
- Chest pain or discomfort

➢ **Pathophysiology:**

Under normal physiological circumstances, oxygen binds to the hemoglobin and forms "oxy-hemoglobin" and thus transports and supplies oxygen to the tissues. However, higher concentrations of carbon monoxide displace oxygen from the hemoglobin due to its high affinity (>200 times than oxygen) and binding with the hemoglobin, forming carboxyhemoglobin or COHb. Since highly metabolic tissues and organs do not receive optimal oxygenation, they undergo anaerobic glycolysis. The end product of the anaerobic glycolysis is lactate. It is acidic and ultimately results in organ failure and death, if not quickly recognized and corrected. Another mechanism of injury is enzymatic derangements at the cellular level, which causes mitochondrial damage and cytotoxicity. Formation of free radicals and the resultant injury is another plausible mechanism of tissue injury. This injury is not only caused by carbon monoxide itself but also has theoretical risks due to treatment with100% oxygen and hyperbaric treatment when used in patients with CO poisoning.

➢ **Laboratory Analysis:**

- Arterial blood gas (ABG)
- Carboxyhemoglobin level (COHb)—Co-oximizer is used in lieu of oximetry
- Clinical symptoms of carbon monoxide poisoning don't correlate with the COHb levels
- Symptoms often ensue at >20-30 parts per million (ppm)

➢ **Treatment:**

- Prevention of CO poisoning is paramount, both in domestic and industrial settings
- Garage door should be left open even when the car is in idle position (especially in cold weather when vehicle is left in idle to warm up the engine)

- Remove the affected individual from the carbon monoxide source and the environment
- Provide 100% oxygen
- Hyperbaric oxygen therapy (hyperbaric chamber)

Stevens-Johnson Syndrome

➢ **Definition and Classification:**

Stevens-Johnson syndrome (SJS) and **Toxic Epidermal Necrolysis (TEN)** are severe idiosyncratic reactions most commonly triggered by medications. Fever and mucocutaneous lesions lead to necrosis and sloughing of the epidermis. SJS and TEN are distinguished chiefly by severity and percentage of the body surface involved. The term "SJS/TEN" Is used interchangeably, and collectively is called "SJS."

- **Stevens-Johnson syndrome:** SJS is a less severe condition in which skin sloughing is limited. There is often a prodrome of systemic inflammatory response syndrome. This may lead to erythematous or purpuric macules and plaques. This is associated with the skin manifestation, which ultimately progresses to epidermal necrosis and skin sloughing. Majority of the patients will have their mucous membranes involved. The sites commonly involved are ocular, oral, and genitalia. There may be more than one site affected by this condition.

➢ **Medications** (Most common culprit medications):
- Anti-gout agents (especially allopurinol)
- Antibiotics (sulfonamide > penicillin > cephalosporin)
- Antipsychotics and anti-epileptics (Dilantin, carbamezepine, lamotrigine, and phenobarbital)
- Analgesics and nonsteroidal anti-inflammatory (NSAID) agents (piroxicam)

➢ **Treatment:**
- Stop the culprit medication
- Provide supportive care, including fluid management

- Transfer to burn unit
- Wound care
- Treatment of the underlying infection with empiric antibiotics as indicated

Lidocaine Toxicity

➤ **Definition:**

Lidocaine is a Class 1-B anti-arrhythmic medication. It is a toxicity that occurs after administration of lidocaine doses in an incremental fashion. The total dose may exceed 1.5 mg/kg. Systemic symptoms have been reported at much lower doses; however, much of the toxicity is dose related.

➤ **Pathophysiology:**

Systemic toxicity is caused by elevated methemoglobin level. Normal methemoglobin level is 1-3%. Elevated levels cause oxidation of the iron atoms, and converts from ferrous to ferric state.

➤ **Etiology:**

Topical instillation to the systemic administration of lidocaine

➤ **Mode of Lidocaine Toxicity:**

- Slow: Occurs with continuous infusion such as IV drips
- Sudden and rapid: Occurs when large doses are used in a short span of time, such as during surgery, liposuction, bronchoscopy

➤ **Clinical Symptoms:**

- Visual disturbances
- Neurological problems, seizures, coma
- Respiratory depression
- Cardiovascular problems

➤ **Treatment:**

- Stop the infusion or instillation
- Symptomatic treatment for the seizures
- Methylene blue works as an oxidizing agent
- Benzodiazepines if witnessed seizures (don't treat prophylactically)

- Supportive care, i.e., cardiovascular and respiratory
- Lipid emulsion administered intravenously binds to the drug, reducing its toxicity
  - **Common Causes of Methemoglobinemia**
    Benzocaine, lidocaine, prilocaine, dapsone; organic nitrites/nitrates:
    amyl nitrate, nitroglycerin, nitroprusside; inorganic nitrates: fertilizers, phenazopyridine; quinones: chloroquine, primaquine, sulfonamides

Calcium Channel Blockers (CCB) Toxicity

➤ **Definition:**
It is quite common to get accidental or intentional poisoning with calcium channel blockers. It is a common antihypertensive medicine.

➤ **Pathophysiology:**
CCB blocks the intracellular shift of calcium and causes toxicity due to relaxation of the smooth muscle. It also causes heart block secondary to delay in atrioventricular (AV) conduction.

➤ **Clinical Features:**
- Bradycardia and advanced heart block (myocardial depression)
- Hypotension
- Generalized weakness
- Confusion
- Respiratory depression

➤ **Treatment:**
- Critical care monitoring and treatment
- Gastric lavage if within two hours of ingestion
- Activated charcoal given once upon initial presentation to every patient
- Hemodialysis is less likely to be helpful, since the majority of the drug is protein bound
- Atropine

- A bolus of 1-2 g (10-20 mL 10%) calcium chloride plus a continuous infusion of 20-40 mg/kg/hr (0.2-0.4 mL/kg/hr 10%)
- Dopamine or norepinephrine for hemodynamic support
- Glucagon 2-5 mg IV over 30-60 seconds, can be repeated every five minutes as needed and continuous infusion can be used
- Insulin infusion (start at 1 unit/hr and maintain 0.5 to I unit/hr)
- Pacemaker (external or transvenous) for advanced heart block
- Amrinone or other phosphodiesterase inhibitor (PDE-I)

Beta-Blockers (BB) Toxicity

➤ **Definition:**

Like calcium channel blockers, beta-blocker toxicity may occur due to inadvertent or suicidal overdose

➤ **Pathophysiology:**

Beta-blockers work by competitively inhibiting the action of circulating catecholamines. It causes multiple metabolic effects and also results in atrioventricular (AV) conduction delay or block

➤ **Clinical Features:**

- Bradycardia Q-T prolongation and advanced heart block (myocardial depression)
- Hypotension
- Confusion, seizures, or coma
- Bronchospasm and respiratory depression

➤ **Treatment:**

- Critical care monitoring and treatment
- Gastric lavage if within two hours of ingestion
- Multiple-dose activated charcoals (MDAC)
- Atropine
- Cardiac pacing

- Inotropic and chronotropic support
- Benzodiazepines for the seizures
- Insulin infusion helps due to its positive inotropic properties
- Glucagon infusion
- Hemodialysis when conventional treatment fails, especially in case of atenolol, sotalol, or nodolol overdose (less protein bound)

Hematologic Disorders

1. Disseminated Intravascular Coagulation (DIC)
2. Thrombotic Thrombocytopenic Purpura (TTP)
3. Hematopoietic Stem Cell (HSC) Transplant Complications
4. Peri-Engraftment Respiratory Distress Syndrome (PERDS)
5. Transfusion-Related Lung Injury (TRALI)
6. Transfusion-Related Circulatory Overload (TACO)
7. Heparin-Induced Thrombocytopenia (HIT)
8. Tumor Lysis Syndrome (TLS)
9. Hypercalcemia
10. Blood Transfusion Strategies in the ICU

Disseminated Intravascular Coagulation (DIC)

➢ **Definition:**

A hematological condition characterized by formation of microthrombi in the bloodstream. This is an exaggerated response secondary to an injurious stimulus, which can be of intrinsic or extrinsic nature, i.e., infections, sepsis, or trauma. As a result, these microthrombi clog up the small blood vessels, compromising the essential blood supply to the organs, which results in organ failure. This process of uncontrolled and unchecked thrombosis results due to overutilization and depletion of the clotting factors. There is an increased tendency to bleed, especially from puncture sites and intravenous sites due to utilization of the factors. Conversely this phenomenon may also lead to thrombosis.

➤ **Laboratory Findings:**

- Increased PT/INR
- Increased PTT
- Increased thrombin time
- Decreased fibrinogen
- Increased fibrinogen degrading or split products (FDP/ FSP), which is caused by:
  - □ Increased breakdown of the clots
  - □ Increased D dimer
  - □ Decreased protein C
  - □ Decreased anti-thrombin III (AT-III)
  - □ Decreased platelets

➤ **Predisposing conditions**

- Sepsis
- Trauma
- Malignancy
- Obstetric complications
- Liver failure
- Vascular anomalies
- DIC score- >5=DIC

Lab		
Platelets	>100	0
	<100	1
	<50	2
Elevated FDP	Mild	0
	Moderate	2
	Strong	3
Prolonged PT	<3 s	0
	3-6 s	1
	>6 S	2
Fibrinogen	>100	0
	<100	1

Thrombotic Thrombocytopenic Purpura (TTP)

➢ **Definition:** A hematological condition characterized by severe thrombocytopenia along with systemic manifestation

➢ **Signs and Symptoms (mnemonic pentad of "FAT RN"):**
   ▪ Fever
   ▪ Anemia (microangiopathic: schistocytes, microspherocytes)
   ▪ Thrombocytopenia
   ▪ Renal failure
   ▪ Neurologic dysfunction

➢ **Etiology**
   ▪ Idiopathic
   ▪ Oral contraceptives
   ▪ Pregnancy
   ▪ Drugs (antiplatelets, i.e., Plavix, cyclosporine, quinine)
   ▪ Infection/sepsis
   ▪ Bone marrow transplant

➢ **Pathogenesis**
   ▪ Platelet aggregation in the microvasculature causing ischemic organ damage
   ▪ Congenital deficiency of ADAMSTS-13 metalloproteinase (involved with the degradation of Von-Will brand factor (vWF)
   ▪ May also be caused by an autoimmune disease

➢ **Treatment**
   ▪ Plasma exchange is the first-line treatment
   ▪ Steroids
   ▪ Immunosuppression
   ▪ Splenectomy can be in refractory cases
   ▪ **DO NOT** transfuse platelets because it worsens the clinical outcomes

Hematopoietic Stem Cell Transplant Complications

➢ **0-30 days (early post-transplant or peri-engraftment period)**

Infectious:
- Candida albicans/glabrata
- Aspergillum
- Bacteria

Noninfectious:
- Peri-engraftment respiratory distress syndrome (PERDS)
- Pulmonary edema
- Diffuse alveolar hemorrhage (DAH)

➤ **30-60 days (early post-engraftment)**

Infection:
- Cytomegalovirus (CMV)
- Pneumocystis jiroveci pneumonia (PJP)
- Respiratory syncytial virus (RSV)
- Bacterial infections
- Aspergillum

Non-infections:
- Graft versus host disease (GVHD)
- Diffuse alveolar hemorrhage (DAH)

➤ **>100 days (late post-transplant)**

Infection:
- Encapsulated bacteria (HIB, S. pneumococcus)

Non-infections:
- Chronic graft versus host disease (GVHD)
- Bronchiolitis obliterans (BO)

Peri-Engraftment Respiratory Distress Syndrome (PERDS)

➤ **Definition:**
Respiratory distress caused by idiopathic pneumonia within 30 days of hematopoietic transplant

➤ **Signs/Symptoms:**
- Diarrhea
- Skin rash
- Fever
- Dysphagia

- Cough
- ➤ **Diagnosis:**
  - CXR shows diffuse infiltrates without an obvious source of infection
- ➤ **Treatment:**
  - Steroids (high dose)

Transfusion-Related Acute Lung Injury (TRALI)

- ➤ **Definition:** Acute respiratory distress or failure, which results soon after transfusion of blood products
  - Occurs 2-4 hours post transfusion
  - Pulmonary edema is noncardiogenic in nature and is primarily secondary to the capillary leak
  - Unresponsive to diuretics, since this is an immune-mediated process
- ➤ **Associated with Transfusion of:**
  - Packed red blood cells (PRBC)
  - Whole blood
  - Fresh frozen plasma (FFP)
  - Platelets
  - Cryoprecipitate
- ➤ **Pathogenesis:**
  - HLA-specific antibodies that react with the donor's white blood cells.
  - These WBCs get trapped in the lung, causing damage and capillary leak.
- ➤ **Incidence:**
  - 1 in 5,000
  - 6% mortality
  - 70% require intubation due to respiratory failure
- ➤ **Treatment:**
  - Supportive care
  - Steroids (animal studies only)
  - Spontaneous resolution 3-4 days, no long-term sequalae

➢ **Subsequent Transfusions:**
- Autologous
- Washed

Transfusion-Associated Circulatory Overload (TACO)

➢ **Definition:**
Acute respiratory failure after transfusion of blood products. This phenomenon occurs due to volume overload rather than the immune-mediated process as in TRALI. It tends to occur in susceptible Individuals such as patients with an underlying coronary artery disease or heart failure.

➢ **Pathogenesis:**
- The mechanism of injury is related to the intravascular volume overload.
- It more commonly occurs in patients with underlying coronary artery disease and associated heart failure.

➢ **Treatment:**
- Stop the infusion of the blood product
- Diuresis as needed and tolerated, which is based on the hemodynamic parameters

Heparin-Induced Thrombocytopenia (HIT)

➢ **Definition:**
A sudden and precipitous drop in the platelet count, usually by fifty percent or more of the baseline platelet count. However, the diagnosis is based purely on clinical grounds, rather than laboratory analysis.

➢ **Classification:**
There are two types of HIT:
- **Type I**
  - Occurs 1-2 days after heparin is initiated
  - Mild thrombocytopenia (platelet >100,000)
  - No thrombosis
  - Nonimmunogenic-mediated phenomenon

- ▫ Caused by the binding of heparin to platelet membrane
- ▫ It is self-limited and resolves within 3-5 days
- **Type 2**
  - ▫ Immune-mediated process
  - ▫ Severe thrombocytopenia (platelets <100,000) or 25% drop from the baseline
  - ▫ Increased risk of thrombosis
  - ▫ Heparin antibodies complex formed with heparin and platelet factor 4
  - ▫ Incidence 1-5%
- ➢ **Diagnosis:**
  - Clinical picture
  - Labs shows sign of platelet aggregation, platelet injury, or positive
  - HIT ELISA
- ➢ **Treatment:**
  - Discontinue heparin (both high molecular as well low molecular weight, i.e., Lovenox) and start alternate medication:
    - ▫ Lepirudin (direct thrombin inhibitor, which is cleared by the kidney)
    - ▫ Argatroban (liver clearance)
    - ▫ Anti-factor ten agents (anti-X agent, i.e., fondaparinux)

Tumor Lysis Syndrome (TLS)

- ➢ **Definition:**

  Tumor lysis syndrome occurs when large numbers of neoplastic cells are killed rapidly, i.e., immediately post chemotherapy in patients with fast growing tumors. It is a potentially lethal condition that may occur during cancer treatment. It is typically associated with hematological and solid organ cancers, i.e., leukemia and lymphomas.

- ➢ **Laboratory:**
  - Hyperkalemia
  - Hypocalcemia

- Hyperuricemia
- Hyperphosphatemia
- High BUN/creatinine
- Lactic acidosis

➢ **Clinical:**
- More common in males
- Young age <25 years
- Concentrated acidic urine
- Volume depletion

➢ **Diagnosis:**
- Clinical picture with known or suspected malignancy
- Lab values in the right clinical context

➢ **Treatment:**
- Aggressive hydration, prior to and post chemotherapy
- Alkaline diuresis
- Allopurinol both for prophylaxis and treatment of TLS
- Hemodialysis in some refractory cases

Hypercalcemia

➢ **Definition:** Serum calcium levels > 11.5 mg/dL (2.9 mmol/L)

➢ **Symptoms:**

1: Symptoms at serum calcium level > 11.5 mg/dL
- CNS: Depression, anxiety, headache, fatigue, and cognitive dysfunction
- GI : Constipation, anorexia, and abdominal pain

2: Symptoms at serum calcium level > 13 mg/dL
- Renal: polyuria, polydipsia, and nocturia (associated with renal insufficiency and renal tubular acidosis)

3: Symptoms at serum calcium level > 15 mg/dL
- Medical emergency, may lead to cardiac arrest and coma

➢ **Causes:**
- Primary hyperparathyroidism is the most common cause of hypercalcemia. Hyperparathyroidism can be caused by parathyroid adenoma (81%), parathyroid hyperplasia

(15%), and parathyroid carcinoma (4%).

- Hypercalcemia of malignancy is the second most common cause of hypercalcemia and is often difficult to manage
- Other conditions associated with hypercalcemia include: MEN I, MEN II, sarcoidosis and other granulomatous diseases, severe secondary hyperparathyroidism, vitamin D intoxication, hyperthyroidism, and immobilization
- Thiazides and lithium therapy

➤ **Treatment:**

Type of treatment is based on the underlying cause of hypercalcemia. The most common treatment modalities include hydration with saline, forced diuresis (furosemide with hydration), IV pamidronate, calcitonin, and in severe cases, hemodialysis may be needed.

Blood Transfusion Strategies in the Critical Care Setting

We often come across a wide range of patient clinical presentation in which blood transfusion is required. There are various approaches to transfuse blood. However, a methodical approach is needed in the critical care environment as the patients are very sick, and any treatment modality will have a positive or negative impact. Generally, two blood transfusion approaches are often utilized in the critical care setting.

➤ **Conservative Transfusion Approach (CTA):**
Transfuse only when hemoglobin drops less than 7gram/dl

➤ **Liberal Transfusion Approach (LTA):**
Transfuse when hemoglobin drops less than 9-10 gram/dl

- *Liberal strategy should be employed in patients who are actively bleeding, i.e., trauma victims, GI bleeding. Patients who have an underlying coronary artery disease will also benefit from keeping the Hb> 10. Liberal approach in the other medical ICU patients poses risks of transfusion-associated reactions, such as TACO, TRALI, etc. Therefore, a rather conservative approach should be employed in this patient population.*

Pregnancy and Critical Care

1. Acute Fatty Liver of Pregnancy (AFLP) or Hepatic Lipidosis of Pregnancy
2. HELLP syndrome
3. Amniotic Fluid Embolism
4. Tocolytic-Induced Pulmonary Edema
5. Hemodynamic and Physiologic Changes During Pregnancy
6. Asthma During Pregnancy

Acute Fatty Liver of Pregnancy (AFLP) "Hepatic Lipidosis of Pregnancy"

➤ **Definition:**

It is a rare albeit, life threatening condition which occurs during the third trimester of pregnancy or in the immediate post-partum period. It is caused by deficiency of the enzyme, which metabolizes fatty acids

➤ **Risk Factors:**
- First pregnancy
- Multiple child births
- Associated with mutation of E474Q gene

➤ **Signs/symptoms:**
- Nausea/vomiting
- RUQ pain
- Jaundice
- Increased LFTs and bilirubin

- Encephalopathy
- ➤ **Labs:**
  - Normal peripheral blood smear
- ➤ **Complications:**
  - Fulminant hepatic failure with encephalopathy
  - Renal failure
  - GI bleed
  - Seizure, coma, death
  - Preeclampsia- 50%
- ➤ **Diagnosis:**
  - Diagnosis made on clinical grounds
  - Liver biopsy is not needed for diagnosis of AFLP
- ➤ **Pathogenesis:**
  - Accumulation of micro-vesicular fat can be seen on biopsy
- ➤ **Treatment:**
  - Supportive care
  - Expedited delivery of the fetus

HELLP Syndrome

- ➤ **Definition:**

  Symptom complex or a triad of:
  - Hemolysis
  - Elevated liver enzymes
  - Low platelets
- ➤ **Differential Diagnosis:**
  - Less elevation of liver enzymes as compared with AFLP
  - Jaundice uncommon
    - *Differential diagnosis: Toxemia of pregnancy, which presents with icterus or elevated bilirubin*

Amniotic Fluid Embolism

- ➤ **Definition:**

  It is a catastrophic syndrome that occurs during pregnancy or

in the postpartum period
- ➤ **Risk Factors:**
  - Advanced maternal age
  - Multiparity
  - Use of uterine stimulants
  - Premature rupture of membranes (PROM)
  - Tumultuous labor
  - Cesarean (C-section)
  - Internal fetal monitoring
- ➤ **Clinical Presentation:**
  - Cardiopulmonary arrest
  - Disseminated intravascular coagulation (DIC)
  - Acute respiratory distress syndrome (ARDS)
  - Diagnosis is based on clinical grounds (diagnosis of exclusion)
- ➤ **Treatment:**
  - Supportive care

Tocolytic-Induced Pulmonary Edema
- ➤ **Definition:**
  Development of respiratory distress or failure in pregnant patients who received tocolytic to inhibit uterine contractions during premature labor
- ➤ **Signs/Symptoms:**
  - Tachypnea
  - Tachycardia
  - Hypoxia with an increased A—a gradient on ABGs
  - Shortness of breath
  - Chest pain
  - Cough
  - Normal EKG and cardiac enzymes
- ➤ **CXR:**
  - Bilateral pulmonary infiltrates
  - Normal heart size

➤ **Pathophysiology:**
- Pulmonary edema >24-48h
- Normal BP
- Increased hydrostatic pressure
- Volume overload

➤ **Risk Factors:**
- Prolonged tocolytic treatment >24-48 hours
- Multiple or twin gestation
- Sepsis
- Preeclampsia
- Vigorous volume resuscitation

➤ **Treatment:**
- Stop tocolysis
- Supportive care, including supplemental oxygen and diuresis
- Magnesium sulfate (causes smooth muscle relaxation)

Hemodynamic and Physiologic Changes During Pregnancy

➤ Increase in O2 consumption
➤ Decreased functional residual capacity (FRC)
- Decreased ERV 40%
- Decreased RV 22%
- Reduction in these parameters results from the elevated diaphragm and is accentuated by the recumbent position

➤ Lower O2 reserve, therefore more susceptibility to hypoxia
➤ Increased minute ventilation
- Increased CO2 leads to an increased respiratory drive
- Increased progesterone levels
- Increased TV from increased rib cage volume displacement
- Respiratory alkalosis: normal pH 7.40-7.47, bicarbonate 18-21

➤ Increased cardiac output by 20-30%, heart rate increased by 10-20 beats/minute, and increased stroke volume
➤ Decreased PVR and increased plasma volume by 35-50% to

a total of 7-8 liters at term

➢ Fetal umbilical pO2 is lower than venous PO2

➢ Increased Factors VII, VIII, IX, and X, increased fibrinogen levels to 350-400mg/dl

Asthma During Pregnancy

➢ Asthma is a bronchoreactive airway disease caused by reversible inflammation of the airways. Asthma can be managed with the same medications that are used in the treatment of asthma in a non-pregnant patient population. However, individual labeling should be checked to review the safety instructions, and risk versus benefit should be weighed before dispensing these medicines to pregnant patients.

➢ *Asthma Action Plan* should be handed to all pregnant asthmatics, as there may be more and often severe asthma exacerbation during the pregnancy. These exacerbations should be treated aggressively, since lack of oxygen during these attacks may lead to fetal hypoxia with potentially devastating outcomes.

➢ Uncontrolled asthma may also exacerbate other medical conditions, such as systemic hypertension and preeclampsia/eclampsia.

Gastroenterology Critical Care

1. Alcoholic Hepatitis
2. MELD Score
3. Adynamic Ileus, Pseudo-Obstruction, Ogilvie Syndrome
4. Hepatorenal Syndrome
5. Pancreatitis
6. Re-feeding Syndrome
7. Nutrition in the ICU
8. Gastrointestinal Bleeding (GI Bleeding)
9. Spontaneous Bacterial Peritonitis (SBP)
10. Severe Clostridium Difficile Colitis (C-Diff)
11. Ischemic Colitis (Mesenteric Artery Ischemia)

Alcoholic Hepatitis

To define severity of the alcoholic hepatitis, currently two models are currently employed:

- ➤ **Maddrey's discriminant function**
  - ▪ DF=4.6*(PT-control)+Bilirubin
  - ▪ If greater than 32, steroids reduce 30-day mortality
- ➤ **Model for end-stage liver disease (MELD)***
  - ▪ Survival probability is based on the following parameters:
    - ▫ INR
    - ▫ Bilirubin
    - ▫ Creatinine

    □   Dialysis frequency
- *High score denotes worst probability of survival*
* UNOS, United Network for Organ Sharing, is an organization that screens and allocates organ donation.

"MELD" SCORE
Model for End-Stage Liver Disease
Scoring Formula:
3.78 (serum bilirubin) + 11.2 (INR) + 9.57 (serum creatinine) + 6.43
➤ Three-month mortality prediction, based on the MELD score:
- 40 or more — 71.3% mortality
- 30–39 — 52.6% mortality
- 20–29 — 19.6% mortality
- 10–19 — 6.0% mortality
- <9 — 1.9% mortality

Adynamic Ileus, Pseudo-Obstruction, Ogilvie Syndrome
➤ **Definition:** It is an acute pseudo-obstruction of the colon
➤ **Diagnosis:** KUB/CT scan
➤ **Clinical:**
- A portion or entire colon may be affected
- Absence of mechanical obstruction, such as tumor
- Normal rectal exam
➤ **Treatment (conservative management):**
- NG tube to suction
- Rectal tube
- Stop medications that can slow gut motility, i.e., narcotics
- Search for and treat the metabolic causes or systemic condition such as hypothyroidism, diabetes (gastroparesis)
- If cecal diameter is >12 cm measured by KUB (abdominal x-ray), colonoscopic decompression or surgical evaluation is indicated

➢ **Contraindicated:**
- Anticholinergic—Reglan
- Erythromycin
- Surgery in refractory cases
- Botox or electrical stimulation (more so for the gastroparesis)

Hepatorenal Syndrome

➢ **Definition:**

It is a condition that is characterized by rapid deterioration of the renal function in patients with liver cirrhosis. This is potentially a life-threatening condition.

➢ **Diagnosis:**
- Liver disease (acute or chronic) with portal hypertension
- Creatinine >1.5 or creatinine clearance <40
- Absence of shock, infection, fluid loss, or nephrotoxic drugs
- Absent GI/renal fluid losses
- <500-mg/d urinary protein excretion in absence of ultrasonographic evidence of parenchymal or obstructive kidney disease
- Absence of improvement in renal function despite discontinuation of diuretics and administration of one- to two-liter fluid bolus

➢ **Prognosis:**

Three-day survival is expected once diagnosis is established

➢ **Treatment:**
- Supportive
- Octreotide (somatostatin analogue)
- Midodrine (alpha-1 adrenergic agonist)
- Hospice should be considered when all treatment modalities fail

Pancreatitis

> **Definition:** It is the inflammation of the pancreas
> **Etiology:** Alcohol, hyperlipidemia (hypertriglyceridemia), drugs (HIV), and certain poisons, i.e., scorpion bite
> **Classification:**
> - **Acute Pancreatitis:** Recent symptoms of abdominal pain along with the specific laboratory findings and/or radio-logical evidence of pancreatic inflammation
> - **Chronic Pancreatitis:** Inflammation occurs over pro-longed period of time resulting in pancreatic damage, most commonly caused by chronic alcohol intake
> - **Hemorrhagic Pancreatitis:** Bleeding in the pancreas
> - **Necrotizing Pancreatitis:** Results in the necrosis of the pancreatic tissue, plus/minus infection
> - **Pancreatic Pseudocyst:** Formation of a cyst, or a cavity filled with either inflammatory fluid or pus
> **Diagnosis:**
> - Clinical, lab, and radiology, i.e., x-ray or CT
> - Lipase is the most specific marker to assess the degree of inflammation and to analyze the trend
> **Treatment:**
> - Nothing orally initially (NPO)
> - Pain control
> - IV fluids
> - Antibiotics, if needed for necrotizing pancreatitis
> - Start oral diet, once patient is stable. Start with clear liquids and continue to monitor their symptoms and lipases to see the trend; if lipase levels are trending up, then keep NPO.
> - If unable to eat, NG feeding is acceptable
>   If there is pseudocyst or necrotizing pancreatitis, then feeding with small-bore tube is recommended. It should be placed beyond the ligament of Treitz.
> - Parenteral feeding with the TPN is recommended if oral tube feeding fails

Re-feeding Syndrome

> ➤ **Definition:** This phenomenon occurs when oral or tube feeding is restarted in patients after prolonged periods of starvation. It is associated with profound electrolyte imbalances and multi-organ failure, which is precipitated in previously malnourished/starved individuals, once the nutrition is started. First noticed after the first World War prisoners who were fed after a prolonged period of starvation.

> ➤ **Laboratory:** There are a host of electrolyte abnormalities associated with the re-feeding syndrome, most specifically hypophosphatemia. Sometimes this may present with normal lab values.

> ➤ **Pathogenesis:** During periods of prolonged malnutrition, the body's metabolism switches from carbohydrates to fats and protein. The end products of fats and proteins are utilized as the primary source of energy expenditure. Hence, the body utilizes less insulin due to lack of carbohydrates. However, upon resuming the normal diet, the metabolic wheel turns towards carbohydrate metabolism and uses it as a source of energy; hence, insulin secretion is increased. This phenomenon causes trans-cellular shift of the extracellular phosphates into the cells, and renders the extracellular milieu rather hypophosphatemic.

> ➤ **Onset and Duration:** Occurs within four days of resumption of regular diet

> ➤ **Clinical Sequalae:** Respiratory failure, heart failure, rhabdomyolysis, renal failure, arrhythmias, coma, seizures, and may result in death

> ➤ **Diagnosis:** High index of suspicion in patients with prolonged malnutrition or under-nutrition (anorexia nervosa) who are re-started on a regular diet through either an enteral or parenteral route, i.e., TPN, PPN
> Phosphate levels are less than 0.5

> ➤ **At-Risk Population:** Anorexia nervosa, cancer, alcoholism, and post op

➤ **Treatment:** IV phosphate infusion with the target phosphate >0.5 mmol and provide supportive care. Start feeding at 25-50% of the estimated caloric needs.

Nutrition in the ICU Setting

➤ **Why Is It Necessary?**
- ↑ Caloric demands in critically ill patients
- ↑ Work of breathing due to underlying pathology:
  □ Sepsis
  □ Fever
  □ Wound healing
  □ Stress hormone release
- ↓ Caloric intake either due to the disease process or simply being NPO
- ↓ Bowel and liver perfusion
- Multiple organ failure
- Medications
- Pre-existing malnutrition

➤ **Consequences of Malnutrition or Under-nutrition:**
Immune System
- Impaired T-cell and B-cell function
- ↓ Liver mass → ↓ acute phase reactants and visceral proteins

Respiratory System
- ↓ Diaphragmatic muscle mass
- ↓ Ventilatory drive
- ↓ Lung parenchymal elastic fibers
- ↓ Surfactant production

➤ **Assessment of Nutritional Status in the ICU:**
Fat Stores
- Triceps skin fold thickness
- BMI = weight (kg)/height (m^2)

Muscle Mass
- Decreased limb circumference

- Decreased 24-hr urinary creatinine

Visceral Proteins (half-life)

- Albumin (18 days)
- Transferrin (8 days)
- Thyroxin-binding pre-albumin (2 days)
- Retinol-binding protein (12 hours)

The most sensitive marker for malnutrition is pre-albumin level.

➢ **How to Determine Energy Expenditure (EE):**

- Rough estimation based on the stress level
- BMI approach
- Harris-Benedict equation (simply use 25 cal/kg/ideal body weight)
- Fick equation
  Indirect calorimetric analysis
  Pulmonary artery catheterization
- British Diabetic Association method

➢ **Assessment of EE Based on Stress Factors:**

Stress Level	Energy Requirement (kcal/kg/day)
Mild	20-30
Moderate	30-40
Severe	40-50

➢ **How to Provide Nutritional Support:**
Enteral

- Orogastric tube (OG-tube)
- Nasogastric tube (NG-tube)
- Nasoduodenal tube (ND-tube)
- Gastrostomy tube (G-tube)
- Jejunal tube (J-tube)

Parenteral

- Peripheral parenteral nutrition (PPN)
- Total parenteral nutrition (TPN)

➤ **Complications of Enteral Feeding:**
Enteral
- Mechanical
  Epistaxis
  Pneumothorax
- Sinusitis
- Diarrhea
- Aspiration
- Abdominal bloating
- Pneumatosis intestinalis and necrosis
- Metabolic
  Glucose intolerance
  Fluid and electrolyte imbalance
  Overfeeding or re-feeding syndrome

➤ **Complications of Parenteral Feeding (TPN):**
- Mechanical
  - Pneumothorax (iatrogenic)
  - Chylothorax
- Line sepsis
- Metabolic
  - Glucose intolerance
  - Hypoglycemia
  - Fluid and electrolyte imbalance
  - Rebound hypoglycemia
  - Overfeeding or re-feeding syndrome
- Abnormal liver function

➤ **Summary:**
- Under-nutrition can occur in mechanically ventilated and critically ill patients due to increased nutritional requirements/metabolic needs, which can impair immunity and respiratory function.
- Prescription of enteral and parenteral nutrition requires estimation of nutritional requirements.
- When feasible, enteral feeding is preferred over parenteral

nutrition due to the relative ease of administration, less likelihood of infection, and lower cost.

- High gastric residuals are allowed, i.e., >400 cc. However, other modalities can be employed to enhance the gut motility, such as Reglan and reducing use of the narcotic medications.

Gastrointestinal Bleeding (GI Bleed)

➤ **Classification:**

- **Upper GI Bleeding**
  - Peptic ulcer disease (PUD)
  - Gastritis or esophagitis
  - Esophageal varices (cirrhosis with portal hypertension)
  - Mallory-Weiss tears, which cause superficial esophageal tears
  - Boerhaave syndrome (perforation of esophagus due to retching/vomiting)
  - Esophageal and gastric cancers
  - Medication, such as anticoagulants, i.e., Coumadin (INR often in the supra-therapeutic range), Pradaxa, NSAIDs, aspirin, and Plavix

- **Lower GI Bleeding**
  - May be caused by rapid upper GI bleed with rapid transit time
  - Diverticulosis/diverticulitis
  - Angiodyplasia/atriovenous malformations (AVM)
  - Colon cancer
  - Inflammatory bowel disease (IBD), Crohn's disease, and ulcerative colitis
  - Infectious causes, Salmonella, Shigella, C-diff colitis
  - Hemorrhoids/fissures
  - Medication such as anticoagulants (often in the supra-therapeutic range), i.e., Coumadin

➤ **Clinical Signs and Symptoms:**
- Hemoptysis (vomiting blood) UGI bleed
- Black, tarry stools or bright red blood per rectum (BRBPR) LGI bleed
- Generalized symptoms related to the blood loss:
  - Fatigue
  - Syncope or near-syncope
  - Shortness of breath
  - Abdominal pain

➤ **Diagnostic Tests:**
- Hemoglobin determination
- Occult blood in stool (guaiac blood)
- Esophagogastroduodenoscopy (EGD) and colonoscopy
- Capsule endoscopy can be performed when colonoscopy is either difficult or nondiagnostic

➤ **Treatment:**
- Keep NPO
- Establish IV access, at least two 16-gauge peripheral lines
- IV fluids until blood products are available
- Blood products, PRBC, platelets, fresh frozen plasma
- Vitamin-K (IV/SC in critically ill patients)
- Cryoprecipitate, factor IIV, i.e., Nova-seven
- Antibiotics (infectious causes)
- Stop the culprit medications (Coumadin, heparin)
- EGD/colonoscopy with therapeutic intent with or without intervention
- Surgery in refractory cases
- Treatment of the underlying cause, i.e., TIPS for portal hypertension
- Proton pump inhibitors (PPI) and octreotide for patients with GI bleed due to liver cirrhosis and associated portal hypertension

Spontaneous Bacterial Peritonitis

➢ **Definition:**

- Infected ascitic fluid without any evidence of intra-abdominal infection. It is most commonly seen in patients with cirrhosis and ascites. Infectious agents include but are not limited to *Escherichia coli, Klebsiella, streptococcal, staphylococcal.*

➢ **Pathophysiology:**

It is usually caused by translocation of the gut-flora. Translocation occurs due to increased hydrostatic pressure, which in conjunction with the decreased oncotic pressure causes translocation of the bacteria across the luminal gradient. This results in increased capillary and tissue leak. Since the ascitic fluid is juxtaposed to the edematous intestines, the bacteria translocate from the intestines to the peritoneal fluid.

➢ **Diagnosis:**

- Positive ascitic fluid gram stain and culture
- Elevated ascitic fluid absolute white cell leukocyte count
- Elevated ascitic fluid lactoferrin
- Serum ascites-albumin gradient (SAAG) >1.1 (helps determine if ascites is caused by elevated portal pressure as in (ESLD) end-stage liver disease

➢ **Signs/Symptoms:**

- Fever
- Abdominal pain/tenderness
- Paralytic or adynamic ileus
- Hypotension
- Hypothermia
- Diarrhea

➢ **Treatment:**

- Broad-spectrum antibiotic therapy
- Cefotaxime or similar third-generation cephalosporin for suspected SBP

- Levofloxacin or norfloxacin
- Surgical intervention, if appropriate (rarely)

Severe Clostridium Difficile (C-Diff) Colitis

➢ **Definition:**
  - It is one of the most common healthcare-acquired infections. This infection is an antibiotic-associated colitis that occurs after normal gut-flora is altered by the use of chronic antibiotic therapy. There is significant morbidity and mortality related to C-diff, especially in the elderly.

➢ **Signs/Symptoms:**
  - Watery diarrhea (10-15 times daily), bloody stools
  - Nausea/vomiting
  - Lower abdominal pain and cramping
  - Low grade fever and leukocytosis (very high WBC count)

➢ **Diagnosis:**
  - Gene test for c-diff is more sensitive
  - Immunoassays for toxins A and B (less sensitive)

➢ **Treatment:**
  - Cessation of the causative antimicrobials
  - Vancomycin (orally)
  - Metronidazole (PO or IV)
  - Combination therapy is recommended in severe c-diff cases, i.e., oral Vancomycin and IV Flagyl (elderly patient with comorbid conditions)

Ischemic Colitis (Mesenteric Artery Ischemia)

➢ **Definition:**
  This is a condition caused by lack of perfusion to the gut vessels

➢ **Pathophysiology:**
  Intestines (both small and large bowel) are supplied by the mesenteric blood vessels. These blood vessels emanate directly from the aorta. Patients who have prolonged hypertension

or peripheral vascular disease are predisposed to the ischemia. It is also common in patients with certain arrhythmias, i.e., atrial fibrillation or flutter. The sluggish, irregular blood flow especially in the absence of anticoagulation on board will result in thromboembolism and gut ischemia.

➢ **Signs/Symptoms** (May be acute or chronic):
- Fever
- Bloody stools
- Abdominal pain after eating
- Nausea/vomiting/diarrhea

➢ **Diagnosis:**
- Clinical suspicion or in presence of an underlying CAD, A-Fib, or PAD
- CT angiogram (mesenteric angiogram) and/or abdominal ultrasound
- Elevated WBC count

➢ **Treatment** (Emergency):
- Thrombolysis
- Surgery for revascularization and removal of the necrotic tissue and end-to-end anastomosis
- Stenting is an alternative approach to surgery in nonsurgical candidates

Critical/Emergent Procedures

1. Central Venous Catheter (CVC)
2. Intraosseous Line (IO)
3. Arterial Line (ART line)
4. Chest Tube/Thoracentesis
5. Paracentesis
6. Lumbar Puncture (LP)
7. Nasogastric/Orogastric Tube (NG/OG tube)
8. Percutaneous Tracheostomy (PERC-TRAC)
9. Cricothyroidotomy (CRIC)
10. Pericardiocentesis

Central Venous Catheter (CVC) or Central Line

CVC is placed in the internal jugular, subclavian, or femoral vein. The procedure is usually performed using aseptic and sterile measures. Consent is required, unless done in an emergency situation.

> **Equipment Required:**
> - The procedure is performed often under ultrasound guidance, especially when performed in a control setting (IJ and S/C route)
> - Central venous kit
> - Sterile drapes, glove, gown, and masks

> **Indications:**
> - Any type of shock, septic, cardiogenic, hypovolemic
> - Blood transfusion in GI bleed and trauma

- Major surgery
- Hemodynamic monitoring, CVP, measurement of cardiac indices by Swan-Ganz catheter

➤ **Complications:**
- Bleeding
- Damage to other structures
- Infection
- Air embolism, if Trendelenburg position is not used during insertion or upon removal of the catheter from the internal jugular vein
- Arrhythmias
- Pneumothorax when inserted in the subclavian or internal jugular vein
- Guide wire can be dislodged or inadvertently left in the vein

Intraosseous Catheter (IO Line)

This is the quickest way of obtaining an intravenous (IV) access

➤ **Indications:**
- In the code situation
- In the field or in an ambulance inserted by paramedics
- Altered level of consciousness
- Respiratory compromise
- Hemodynamic instability

➤ **Equipment:**
- There is special equipment needed for the IO insertion
- "EZ IO" (multiple uses)
- There is a single-use portable push kind

➤ **Anatomical Site:**
- **Tibial access**
  One inch medial and below the medial aspect of the tibial tuberosity
- **Contraindications for tibial access:**
  - Fracture

- □ Previous orthopedic procedure in the anatomical vicinity
- □ Infection at the insertion site
- □ Inability to localize the anatomical landmarks due to trauma or surrounding tissues
- **Iliac crest**
  - □ Superior iliac crest
- **Proximal humerus head**
  - □ The arm should be bent 90 degrees angle at the elbow, and the hand is placed on the umbilicus in a supine position patient. Palpate the mid-shaft humerus and continue palpating upwards towards the humeral head, at the great tubercle. Insert the line in the humeral head.

➤ **Complications:**
- Bleeding
- Infection, especially when attempted in the field
- Damage to the surrounding structures

Arterial Line (A-Line)

➤ **Indications:**

This is done to access the artery for determination of hemodynamic status and frequent arterial blood gases

➤ **Anatomical Sites:**
- Radial artery at the wrist
- Brachial artery in the antecubital fossa
- Axillary artery on the anterior shoulder
- Femoral artery

Chest Tube/Thoracentesis

➤ **Indications:**
- Pleural effusion
- Empyema
- Hemothorax

- Pneumothorax
➤ **Anatomical Site:**
  - Fourth intercostal space, anterior or mid-axillary line
  - Second intercostal space, mid-clavicular line in an emergency situation
  - Ultrasound is used to localize the area of most fluid
➤ **Complications:**
  - Pneumothorax
  - Bleeding
  - Infection

Paracentesis
➤ **Indications:**
Presence of ascites; for diagnostic/therapeutic purposes
➤ **Anatomical Site:**
It is performed with a specialized needle on the anterior abdominal wall, usually on the flanks to avoid injury to the urinary bladder. It is performed under ultrasound guidance.
➤ **Complications:**
  - Bleeding
  - Peritonitis
  - Hemodynamic collapse, if large volume paracentesis is performed
  - Concurrent albumin is infused just before or during large volume paracentesis is performed

Lumbar Spinal Puncture (LP)
➤ **Procedure:**
It is performed at midline in the intervertebral disc space, between posterior superior and iliac supine. This could be performed while the patient is in the lateral position or sitting up on a bed, completely bent over for maximal flexion of spine.
➤ **Indications:**
LP is performed to remove cerebrospinal fluid (CSF) for

diagnostic or therapeutic purposes. Most commonly per-formed for the diagnosis of infections, i.e., meningitis or cancer. It can also be performed when there is increased in-tracranial pressure and the removal of the CSF is indicated for therapeutic reasons. Chemotherapeutic agents can also be administered, intrathecally for the specific cancer treatment.

➤ **Complications:**
- Bleeding/hematoma
- Infection
- CSF leak
- Meningitis
- Death

Nasogastric/Orogastric Tube (NG/OG tube)

➤ **Indications:**
- Tube feeding
- Medication
- Prevent aspiration
- X-ray confirmation is required

➤ **Complications:**
- May inadvertently be placed in the lung

➤ **Contraindications:**
- Boerhaave syndrome
- CSF leak due to fracture of the cribriform bone
- Facial trauma
- Lye or alkali ingestion

Percutaneous Tracheostomy

➤ **Procedure:**
It is performed by making a midline anterior neck incision be-tween second and third tracheal ring. This usually requires two physicians. The first surgeon performs the surgical procedure, while the second physician manages the airway and performs the bronchoscopy and guides the anatomical landmarks.

> **Complications:**
  - Bleeding, especially if innominate vein is severed during the procedure; therefore, avoid very "low approach"
  - Damage to cartilage and surrounding neck structures
  - Esophageal rupture
  - Hypoxia
> **Indication:**
  - Prolonged endotracheal intubation, to prevent tracheomalacia and vocal cord damage
  - Emergency situations, when conventional methods of intubation have failed
  - After radical head and neck dissection

Cricothyroidotomy

> **Procedure:**

Similar to tracheotomy, cricothyroidotomy is performed mostly under *dire straits*. It is often indicated in trauma or burns setting when conventional methods to establish an airway have failed. The incision is made between the cricoid and thyroid cartilage. Only oxygenation can be performed using "Y" tubing. This is performed by jet insufflations, where inspiration is given for one second, followed by closure of the tube for four seconds, to allow time for exhalation. This is only a temporary solution, as this method can provide oxygen only and there is no ventilation. Lack of proper ventilation, therefore, results in the buildup of carbon dioxide and ultimately leads to ventilatory failure from respiratory and metabolic acidosis. Once cricothyroidotomy is performed and there is oxygen flow, definite airway should be attempted as soon as possible.

Pericardiocentesis

> **Indications:**

Removal of fluid from the pericardial sac, either therapeutically such as in case of pericardial tamponade or for diagnostic purposes

➢ **Types of Pericardiocentesis:**
  ▪ Percutaneous (most commonly performed)
  ▪ Surgical

➢ **Procedure:**
Percutaneous procedure is often performed at the bedside or in a cardiac catheterization lab. Echocardiography is performed prior to the procedure to assess the location and the size of the effusion. INR or prothrombin time (PT) and CBC are done prior to the procedure to assess for risk of bleeding and check baseline hemoglobin levels. Ultrasound or fluoroscopy guidance is needed for the procedure. Continuous EKG monitoring is performed throughout the procedure to evaluate for myocardial injury. The needle is appropriately positioned to minimize the risk of myocardial injury.

The substernal or subxiphoid approach is the most commonly employed technique. The site is prepared in a sterile fashion, and topical anesthetic, i.e., lidocaine, is infiltrated into the skin and subcutaneous tissue to achieve an optimal numbness of the insertion site. After localizing the site and determination of the shortest distance from the skin to the pericardial fluid, the needle is inserted and directed towards the left shoulder region at a 45-degree angle. A continuous suction is applied to the cylinder of the syringe by pulling back. This applies a negative pressure and assures the needle has reached the pericardial sac and is not pushed any further, which may cause damage. The patient remains relatively propped up during the procedure to allow for the gravity-based drainage. Once in the pericardial sac, a soft wire is inserted through the needle into the pericardial sac. Subsequently, a catheter is inserted over the guide-wire using the Seldinger technique. A stopcock is attached to the end of the catheter. The pericardial fluid is drained either intermittently or continuously, depending on the clinical objective or the underlying pathology.

➢ **Complications:**
- Cardiac lacerations
- Arrhythmia
- Bleeding
- Pneumothorax
- Infection
- Death

Medical Ethics

Autonomy: Patient has the ultimate right to refuse or choose their treatment

(*Voluntas aegroti suprema lex*) If the patient is incapacitated due to reversible or irreversible medical condition and can't make decisions, then this tenet is decided by the "power of attorney" (POA), surrogate decision maker, or a court-appointed guardian

Beneficence: To act in the best Interest of the patient (*Salus aegroti suprema lex*)

Nonmaleficence: "First, do no harm" (*primum non nocere*), from the *Hippocratic Oath*

Justice: Concerns the distribution and utilization of health resources, and the decision of who gets what treatment (system of triage emerged for this tenet)

Abbreviations

A Fib: Atrial Fibrillation
A Flutter: Atrial Flutter
ABG: Arterial Blood Gas
ACLS: Advanced Cardiac Life Support
ACS: Acute Coronary Syndrome
ADH: Antidiuretic Hormone
AFLP: Acute Fatty Liver of Pregnancy
AIDS: Acquired Immune Deficiency Syndrome
ALI: Acute Lung Injury
A-Line: Intra-arterial Line
ALS: Amyotrophic Lateral Sclerosis
Ambu: Mask valve bag, designed to deliver ventilation and oxygenation
ANA: Antinuclear Antibody
AP: Anterior Posterior
ARDS: Acute Respiratory Distress Syndrome
ARF: Acute Renal Failure
ATLS: Advanced Trauma Life Support
BAL: Bronchoalveolar Lavage
BB: Beta-Blockers
BiPAP: Bi-Level Positive Airway Pressure
BP: Blood Pressure
BSA: Body Surface Area
CABG: Coronary Artery Bypass Graft
CAD: Coronary Artery Disease

CAP: Community-Acquired Pneumonia
CCRT: Chronic Renal Replacement Therapy
CCB: Calcium Channel Blockers
CF: Cystic Fibrosis
CHF: Congestive Heart Failure
CI: Cardiac Index
cm: Centimeter
CMS: Center for Medicare/Medicaid Services
CO: Carbon Monoxide
CO: Cardiac Output
CO2: Carbon Dioxide
COPD: Chronic Obstructive Pulmonary Disease
CPAP: Continuous Positive Airway Pressure
CRT: Cardiac Resynchronization Therapy
CSA: Central Sleep Apnea
CSF: Cerebrospinal Fluid
CT: Computed Tomography
CTEPH: Chronic Thrombo Embolic Pulmonary Hypertension
CVA: Cerebrovascular Accident (stroke)
CVC: Central Venous Catheter
CVD: Congenital Valvular Disease
CVP: Central Venous Pressure
CVVH: Continuous Veno-Venous Hemofiltration
CXR: Chest X-Ray
DCS: Decompression Syndrome
D-DIMER: Fibrin Degradation Dimer
DIC: Disseminated Intravascular Coagulation
DVT: Deep Venous Thrombosis
EF: Ejection Fraction
EKG: Electrocardiogram
EMG: Electromyography
ESR: Erythrocyte Sedimentation Rate
ETT: Endotracheal Tube
EZ PAP: Easy Positive Airway Pressure

FFP: Fresh Frozen Plasma

FiO2: Fractionated Oxygen Levels

GBS: Guillain-Barré Syndrome

GCS: Glasgow Coma Scale

GFR: Glomerular Filtration Rate

GI: Gastrointestinal

GNR: Gram Negative Rods

GPC: Gram Positive Cocci

G-Tube: Gastric Tube or PEG tube

HCAP: Healthcare-Acquired Pneumonia

HD: Hemodialysis

HELLP: Hemolysis Elevated Liver Enzymes and Low Platelets

HgbA1C: Glycosylated Hemoglobin Levels

HIT: Heparin-Induced Thrombocytopenia

HIV: Human Immune Deficiency Virus

HTN: Hypertension

HUS: Hemolytic Uremic Syndrome

IABP: Intra-Aortic Balloon Pump

ICP: Intracranial Pressure

ICU: Intensive Care Unit

IJ: Internal Jugular

IO: Intraosseous

IPF: Idiopathic Pulmonary Fibrosis

IPPV: Intermittent Positive Pressure Ventilation

IS: Incentive Spirometry

ITP: Idiopathic Thrombotic Purpura

IV: Intravenous

IVC: Inferior Vena Cava filter

IVIG: Intravenous Immune Globulin

J-tube: Jejunal Tube, placed beyond the ligament of Treitz

JVD: Jugular Venous Distension

KD/HD: Kidney Dialysis/Hemodialysis

KUB: Kidney, Ureter, Bladder view (abdominal x-ray)

LBBB: Left Bundle Branch Block

LDH: Lactate Dehydrogenase
LFT: Liver Function Tests
LMA: Laryngeal Mask Airway
LOC: Level of Consciousness
LOS: Length of Stay
LVAD: Left Ventricular Assist Device
LVEDP: Left Ventricular End Diastolic Pressure
MAOI: Monoamine Oxidase Inhibitor
MAP: Mean Arterial Pressure
MEq: Milli-Equivalent
MFS: Miller Fisher Syndrome
MI: Myocardial Infarction
MM: Multiple Myeloma
mm: millimeters
MRI: Magnetic Resonance Imaging
MRSA: Methicillin Resistant Staphylococcus Aureus
MSSA: Methicillin Sensitive Staphylococcus Aureus
NCS: Nerve Conduction Studies
NCSE: Nonconvulsive Status Epilepticus
NG-Tube: Nasogastric Tube
NIF: Negative Inspiratory Force
NM: Nuclear Medicine
NPO: Nothing Per Oral (food and water restriction)
NPPE: Negative Pressure Pulmonary Edema
NSTEMI: Non-ST Segment Elevation Myocardial Infarction
O2: Oxygen
OG tube: Orogastric tube
OSA: Obstructive Sleep Apnea
P/F RATIO: Ventilation/Fractionated Oxygen Ratio
paO2: Partial Pressure of Oxygen (determined by the ABG)
pCO2: Partial Pressure of Carbon Dioxide
PCWP: Pulmonary Capillary Wedge Pressure
PE: Pulmonary Embolism
PEA: Pulseless Electrical Activity

PEEP: Positive End Expiratory Pressure
PFT: Pulmonary Function Test
PICC: Peripherally Inserted Central Catheter
PIP: Peak Inspiratory Pressure
PPI: Proton Pump Inhibitors
PPlat: Plateau Pressure
PPN: Peripheral Parenteral Nutrition
PRBC: Packed Red Blood Cell
PROM: Premature Rupture Of Membranes
PVR: Pulmonary Vascular Resistance
RA: Right Atrium
RAP: Right Atrial Pressure
ROSC: Return of Spontaneous Circulation
RSBI: Rapid Shallow Breathing Index
RSV: Respiratory Syncytial Virus
RV: Right Ventricle
RVR: Rapid Ventricular Response
RVSP: Right Ventricular Systolic Pressure
S/C: Subclavian
ScVO2: Mixed Venous Oxygen Saturations
SARS: Systemic Airway Respiratory Syndrome
SIRS: Systemic Inflammatory Response Syndrome
SLE: Systemic Lupus Erythematosus
ST: ST Segment
STEMI: ST Segment Elevation Myocardial Infarction
SVR: Systemic Vascular Resistance
TACO: Transfusion-Associated Circulatory Overload
TBI: Traumatic Brain Injury
TEE: Transesophageal Echocardiography
TIA: Transient Ischemic Attack
TIPS: Transjugular Intrahepatic Porto Systemic Shunt
TPN: Total Parenteral Nutrition
TRALI: Transfusion-Related Acute Lung Injury
VTE: Venous Thromboembolism (refers to DVT/PE)

TTP: Thrombotic Thrombocytopenic Purpura
TV: Tidal Volume
UTI: Urinary Tract Infection
VAP: Ventilator-Associated Pneumonia
VBG: Venous Blood Gas
VFIB: Ventricular Fibrillation
VIDD: Ventilator-Associated Diaphragmatic Dysfunction
VQ Scan: Ventilation/Perfusion Scan
VTACH: Ventricular Tachycardia
WM: Waldenstrom's Macroglobulinemia
X-R: X-ray

References

Kumar, Abbas and Fausto. *Robbins and Cotran Pathologic Basis of Disease*, 7th edition.

Gabrielli, Layon, Yu. *Civetta, Taylor and Kirby's Critical Care*, 5th edition.

Irwin and Rippes. *Intensive Care Medicine*, 6th edition.

Loscalzo. *Harrison's Pulmonary and Critical Care Medicine*.

Kasper, Braumwald, Fauci, Hauser, Longo, Jameson. *Harrison's Principles of Internal Medicine*, 16th edition.

ICU book by Paul Marino.

Uptodate (various topics).

J Neurosurg 1994 Jan;80(1):46-50.

J Neurosurg 1995 Dec;83(6):949-62.

Emerg Med J 2001 Nov;18(6):453-7.

JAMA 2004 Mar 17;291(11):1350-7.

Stroke 2002 Jan;33(1):136-40.

J Neurosurg 1993 Sep;79(3):354-62.

Anesthesiology 1978 Sep;49(3):159-64.

Lancet 2005 Jun 21;365(9475):1957-9.

Cochrane Database Syst Rev 2000;(2):CD000196.

Lancet 1987 Jan 10;1(8524):66-9.

Am J Physiol 1988 Aug;255(2 Pt 2):H343-6.

Adams et al 1986: In post-operative multiple trauma patients, no difference in complication rates, average caloric intake, and nitrogen balance between jejunostomy feeding vs. TPN.

Moore et al 1989. 75 patients with abdominal trauma, post-laparotomy Rate of major infections: TPN (20%) > Enteral (3%).

Kudsk et al 1992. In trauma patients, jejunostomy group (vs. TPN) had fewer episodes of pneumonia, intra-abdominal abscess, and line-related sepsis.

Cerra et al 1988. In septic, hypercatabolic patients, no difference in outcome.

Whitesides TE, Haney TC, Morimoto K, Harada H. Tissue pressure measurements as a determinant for the need of fasciotomy. *Clin Orthop Relat Res.* Nov-Dec 1975;43-51.

Lemierre's foundation (Justin E. Rodgers Foundation).

Harrigan MR (1996). "Cerebral salt wasting syndrome: a review." *Neurosurgery* 38 (1): 152–60.

Evaluating Traditional Prognostic Measures in Patients Undergoing Hypothermia After Cardiac Arrest. John C. O'Horo, M.D.,1 Mihail Andreev, M.D., 2 Wael Hassan, M.D.,1 and Asif Anwar, M.D., M.S., FCCP3.*

Cytokines and cell adhesion molecules associated with high-intensity eccentric exercise. L.L. Smith, A. Anwar. M. Fragen, C. Ronato, R. Johnson, D. Holbert. European Journal of Applied Physiology (2000) 82: 61-67 2000.

ARDS Berlin Criteria *JAMA.* 2012;307(23):2526-2533.

ATLS, by American College of Surgeons.

Johannigman et al. Surgery 2000.

ARDSnet study.

Undersea Hyperb Med. 2012 Mar-Apr;39(2):657-65.

i. Symptoms of carbon monoxide poisoning do not correlate with the initial carboxyhemoglobin level. Hampson NB, Dunn SL; UHMCS/CDC CO Poisoning Surveillance Group.

ii. Center for Hyperbaric Medicine, Virginia Mason Medical Center, Seattle, Washington, USA.

Anthony S. Fauci, Eugene Braunwald, Dennis L. Kasper, Stephen L. Hauser, Dan L. Longo, J. Larry Jameson, Joseph Loscalzo, *Harrison's Manual of Medicine* -17th edition 2009 - ISBN: 978-0-07-170200-3.

- www.clevelandclinicmeded.com/medicalpubs/ diseasemanagement/endocriogy.
- /hypercalcemia/.
- Skjønsberg H, Hartmann A, Fauchald P. [Acute renal failure caused by hypercalcemia]. Tidsskr. Nor. Laegeforen. 2001 Jun 10;121(15):1781–3.
- de Torrente A, Berl T, Cohn PD, Kawamoto E, Hertz P, Schrier RW. Hypercalcemia of acute renal failure: Clinical significance and pathogenesis. AJ of Med. 1976 Jul;61(1):119–23.
- Taniegra ED. Hyperparathyroidism. Am Fam Phys. 2004 Jan 15;69(2):333–9.
- 6: Mundy GR, Oyajobi B, Padalecki S, Sterling JA.
- Hypercalcemia of Malignancy. *Clinical Endocrine Oncology* [Internet]. Blackwell Publishing, Ltd; 2009 [cited 2012 Oct 15]. p. 561–6. Available from: http:// onlinelibrary.wiley.com/doi/10.1002/9781444300222. ch77/summary.

Joint National Committee on Prevention, Detection, Evaluation, and Treatment of High Blood Pressure. Sixth Report. Arch Intern Med 1997; 157: 2413–46.

National High Blood Pressure Education Program. The seventh report of the Joint National Committee on prevention, detection, evaluation, and treatment of high blood pressure. Bethesda (MD): Dept. of Health and Human Services, National Institutes of Health, National Heart, Lung, and Blood Institute; 2004. NIH Publication No. 04–5230.

THE LANCET • Vol 356 • July 29, 2000. Division of Cardiology, Department of Medicine, Weill Medical College of Cornell University, New York Presbyterian Hospital, New York, NY, USA (C J Vaughan MRCPI).

Finnerty FA. Hypertensive encephalopathy. Am J Med 1972; 52: 672–78.

Anthony S. Fauci, Eugene Braunwald, Dennis L. Kasper, Stephen L. Hauser, Dan L. Longo, J. Larry Jameson, Joseph Loscalzo. *Harrison's Manual of Medicine* 17th edition 2009 - ISBN: 978-0-07-170200-3.

Shayne PH, Pitts SR. Severely increased blood pressure in the emergency department. *Ann Emerg Med.* Apr 2003;41(4):513-29.

Rhoades R, Planzer R. *Human Physiology.* 3rd ed. Fort Worth: Saunders College Publishing; 1996.

Zampaglione B, Pascale C, Marchisio M, Cavallo-Perin P. Hypertensive urgencies and emergencies. Prevalence and clinical presentation. *Hypertension.* Jan 1996;27(1):144-7.

Pancioli AM. Hypertension management in neurologic emergencies. *Ann Emerg Med.* Mar 2008;51(3 Suppl):S24-7.

Anderson CS, Huang Y, Wang JG, Arima H, Neal B, Peng B, et al. Intensive blood pressure reduction in acute cerebral haemorrhage trial (INTERACT): a randomised pilot trial. *Lancet Neurol.* May 2008;7(5):391-9.

Anthony S. Fauci, Eugene Braunwald, Dennis L. Kasper, Stephen L. Hauser, Dan L. Longo, J. Larry Jameson, Joseph Loscalzo. *Harrison's Manual of Medicine* 17th edition 2009 - ISBN: 978-0-07-170200-3.

I. Nolan CR III, Linas SL: Malignant hypertension and other hypertensive crises. In: *Diseases of the Kidney*, 5th edition. Edited by Schrier RW, Gottschalk CW. Boston, Little, Brown and Co.,1993, pp 1555-1643.

Chagriya Kitiyakara and Nicolas J. Guzman. Division of Nephrology and Hypertension. Georgetown University Medical Center, Washington, DC.

Hsu, CY. Does Non-Malignant Hypertension Cause Renal Insufficiency? Evidence-Based Perspective. Current Opinions in Nephrological Hypertension, 11(3):267-72.

Nadar S, et al. Echocardiographic Changes in Patients with Malignant Phase

Hypertension: The West Birmingham Malignant Hypertension Register. Journal of Human Hypertension, 19(1):69-75.

Voights, Mary Beth: State of Illinois Trauma Nurse Specialist Program, Trauma in Pregnancy, January 2009.

LaMont, J Thomas. Clinical Manifestations and Diagnosis of Clostridium Difficile Infection in Adults: 2012 UpToDate.com, June 11, 2012.

Kelly, Ciaran P and J Thomas LaMont: Treatment of Clostridium Difficile Infection in Adults: 2012 UpToDate.com, July 18, 2012.

Runyon, Bruce A: Diagnosis of Spontaneous Peritonitis: 2012 UpToDate.com, October 10, 2012.

Roger VL, Go AS, Lloyd-Jones DM, et al. Heart disease and stroke statistics—2011 update: A report from the American Heart Association. *Circulation*. 2011;123(4):e18–e209. [Epub Dec. 15, 2010.]

American Heart Association (June 16, 2011). Implantable Medical Devices for Heart Failure. In American Heart Association. Retrieved Nov. 20, 2011 from www.heart.org/HEARTORG/Conditions/HeartFailure/ PreventionTreatmentofHeart Diseases

Slaughter, MD, Rogers, JG, Milano CA, et al. Advanced heart failure treated with continuous-flow left ventricular assist device. N Eng J Med. 2009;361(23):2241–2251.

Kato TS, Schulze PC, Yang J, et al. Pre-operative and post-operative risk factors associated with neurologic complications in patients with advanced heart failure supported by a left ventricular assist device. J Heart Lung Transplant. 2012;31(1):1–8. [Epub Oct. 8, 2011.]

Patel P, Williams JG, Brice JH. Sustained ventricular fibrillation in an alert patient: Preserved hemo-dynamics with a left ventricular assist device. Prehosp Emerg Care. 2011;15(4):533–536. [Epub Aug 1. 2011.]

Brenyo A, Rao M, Koneru S, et al. Risk of mortality for ventricular arrhythmia in ambulatory LVAD patients. J Cardiovasc Electrophysiol. Nov. 14, 2011.

Blood transfusion in elderly patients with acute MI. Wen-Chih Wu, MD, NEJM, Vol 345, No. 17. Oct 25, 2001.

Nephrotoxic effects in high-risk patients undergoing angiography. Peter Aspelin, MD. NEJM/ Vol.348, No.6-491.

Hauser SC. Vascular diseases of the gastrointestinal tract. In: Goldman L, Schafer AI, eds. Cecil Medicine. 24th ed. Philadelphia, PA: Saunders Elsevier; 2011:chap 145.

Richards DB, Knaut AL. Drowning. In: Marx JA, Hockberger RS, Walls RM, et al, eds. Rosen's Emergency Medicine: Concepts and Clinical Practice. 7th ed. Philadelphia, PA: Mosby Elsevier; 2009: chapter 143.

American College of Emergency Physicians, reference materials.

Center for Disease Control, reference materials.